Oral Contraception
in Perspective

Oral Contraception in Perspective

Thirty years of clinical experience with the pill

by A. D. G. Gunn

with contributions by
R. B. Greenblatt, J. Guillebaud,
D. M. Potts and F. Riphagen

Foreword by Egon Diczfalusy

The Parthenon Publishing Group

International Publishers in Science & Technology

Casterton Hall, Carnforth,
Lancs, LA6 2LA, UK

120 Mill Road, Park Ridge,
New Jersey, USA

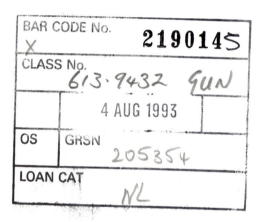
Published in the UK and Europe by
The Parthenon Publishing Group Ltd.
Casterton Hall
Carnforth, Lancs. LA6 2LA   ISBN: 1-85070-150-4

Published in North America by
The Parthenon Publishing Group Inc.
120 Mill Road
Park Ridge
New Jersey, NJ, USA   ISBN: 0-940813-03-3

The Contributors

E. Diczfalusy
Professor of Reproductive
  Endocrinology
Karolinska Institute
Stockholm, Sweden

R. B. Greenblatt
Professor Emeritus
The Medical School of
  Georgia
Augusta
Georgia, USA

J. Guillebaud
Medical Director
The Margaret Pyke Centre
London, England

A. D. G. Gunn
Director of Student Health
The University of Reading
Reading, England

D. M. Potts
President
Family Health
  International
Research Triangle Park
North Carolina, USA

F. Riphagen
Director
The International Health
  Foundation
Brussels, Belgium

Contents

Foreword   9

Introduction
Chemistry in the Mexican jungle   11

Chapter 1
Contraception in history   13

Chapter 2
Hormone research   23

Chapter 3
The first use of hormonal contraception   29

Chapter 4
The impact of social changes due to the pill   39

Chapter 5
The 'image' of the pill – a remarkable social change   45

Chapter 6
The pill and women's health   63

Chapter 7

The evolution of the pill and the surveillance of its effects   69

Chapter 8

The mechanism of the pill   75

Chapter 9

The pill in perspective   85

Chapter 10

The pill and the future   115

Epilogue

The state of the art   125

Index   150

Foreword

William Faulkner says somewhere that 'the past is never dead; it is not even past'. Thirty years ago, in September 1956, I was 'present at the creation' — when I attended the 13th Annual Laurentian Hormone Conference at Mont Tremblant. This series of conferences was created by Gregory Pincus, our 'Goody', and at this particular occasion John Rock, Celso Ramon Garcia and Gregory Pincus, in a paper of historical dimensions, described the first clinical studies on oral contraceptives under the unpretentious title 'Synthetic progestins in the normal human menstrual cycle' (*Rec. Prog. Horm. Res.*, **13**, 323, 1957). At that time (like today), contraception and fertility regulation was a controversial issue touching sensitive nerves and issues central to the human condition. At that time (like today), there was considerable disagreement on the likely impact of family planning on population growth and economic development. What is then the change? It is both significant and irreversible. Since 1956 the world population doubled, from 2.5 billions to 5 billions, and family planning became one of the major concerns of a large number of developing country governments and specialised agencies of the United Nations, such as the World Health Organisation (WHO) and the Family Planning Association (UNFPA). It is also realised today that increased and expanded research efforts are required — beyond the pill — to develop a much wider variety of safe and improved fertility-regulating agents to suit the individual situation, the socio-economic condition and the cultural and religious values of different couples. However, it is obvious that steroidal contraception came to stay with us for a long time; indeed, oral contraceptives are used by some sixty million women today.

In retrospect it seems clear that the introduction of steroidal contraception thirty years ago was indeed a new departure in the history of mankind and a major revolution from the scientific, public health and social points of view. It was, therefore, both appropriate and timely that the Parthenon Publishing Group decided to mark this occasion by publishing this volume. I was delighted to read the different chapters by Derek Gunn, Robert Greenblatt, John Guillebaud, Malcolm Potts and Fritz Riphagen, and I hope, and indeed expect, that a large number of my colleagues will be too.

Time is flying, and eighty years have passed since George Santayana remarked that 'fanaticism consists in redoubling your efforts when you have forgotten your aim', and it is sad to see that fanaticism, rather than critical reflection, became a characteristic feature of our times. Reading the various chapters of this book provided me with a greatly needed opportunity for some reflection on where we stand and where we intend to go in a field of critical importance.

Egon Diczfalusy

Stockholm, September 1986

Introduction:
Chemistry in the Mexican Jungle

Advances in medicine are rarely in its practice, since that is an art; true steps forward are achieved only as a result of advances in technology. Christian Barnard could perform the first transplantation of a human heart only because anesthetics had developed life-support apparatus to maintain the human body alive while he undertook the incisions and the sutures. Howard Florey's medical staff could administer the first-ever doses of penicillin only because Chain and his colleagues had developed techniques for its distillation, albeit then in microscopic quantities insufficient to save the life of the first patient to receive it. So it was also for the oral contraceptive —the 'pill' — for without the maverick enthusiasm in the early 1940s of an American organic chemist, Russell E. Marker, who developed a technique for extracting the essence of a species of Mexican yam and then synthesising from it the female sex hormone progesterone in such prodigious quantities that it became readily available for widespread medical use and research, the 'pill' would perhaps never have been invented. At the time that Russell Marker was developing his technique, the only source of progesterone that was available was from a complicated extract from pregnant mares' urine and it cost $80 an ounce to make. Within less than a year Marker had made three kilograms of it from a vegetable source that grew wild in the jungle near Vera Cruz in Mexico. He made it in the rented laboratory of a friend and astonished the world's leading pharmaceutical firms by making readily available in bulk the first synthesised human sex hormone. His technology in extracting the chemical substance diosgenin (which has exactly the same steroid nucleus as cholesterol but one different side-chain) and in a series of simple but exceedingly brilliant processes degrading two of the diosgenin rings until it was transformed chemically into the sex hormone progesterone was what led, literally, to the possibility of inventing the pill.

Six years later Marker left the company he had founded in Mexico City and gave up chemistry abruptly and totally, dedicating himself for the next thirty years to commissioning local copies of European silver antiques. No public recognition was ever given to this remarkable chemist until 1969 when the Mexican Chemical Society presented him with a special award — a silver tray — at an international symposium on steroids. The man whose work led to a whole new era of medical care, treatment, life-saving, and the liberation of modern generations of women died, unhonoured, in 1984.

What was the origin of the pill? Was it a thoughtless experiment on uninformed women, or was it the most rational method of controlling fertility yet devised? Has it led to an epidemic of heart disease, cancer and strokes or has it been a miraculous life-saver? Are people too pessimistic or too naive about the pill and its effects? Did oral contraceptives cause the sexual revolution, or did they just happen to be a well illuminated symbol? Did the Vatican halt its spread, or has the pill undermined the Church? Did the maverick chemist receive a silver tray for enslaving or liberating half the human race? These are the questions this book attempts to answer.

Chapter 1

Contraception in History

We did not always need artificial contraception. The handful of hunter-gatherer communities which survived into the modern world have stable populations. Like our cousins, the apes, we are amongst the slowest breeding animals known.

Paleolithic women had a life expectancy of thirty years and from late puberty to the menopause it was lactation that spaced their ovulation. Hunter-gatherer tribes breastfed their children for several years. Equally important, they fed their infants several times an hour throughout the day and slept with them at night, all of which promotes the suppression of ovulation.

Lactation was Nature's contraceptive until the development of agriculture and the prospect of a settled, instead of a nomadic, lifestyle began to unravel the machinery evolution had build up so slowly. There is an assumption that the cradle of civilisation for man was in the Middle East. Certainly, the climatic conditions and the environment of the time suggest that within the area bounded by modern Iran, Iraq, Syria, the Lebanon, Jordan, Israel and Egypt tribal life became more settled some 20000 years ago. Eventually, through the use of writing, trade, horticulture, animal husbandry and crafts, patterns of breastfeeding changed and fertility rose. Although these changes were not understood, rational (and sometimes irrational) medical interventions became one of the hallmarks of civilisation. Archaeologists have unearthed the earliest of written evidence to indicate that medical intervention was increasingly practised throughout the later millennia.

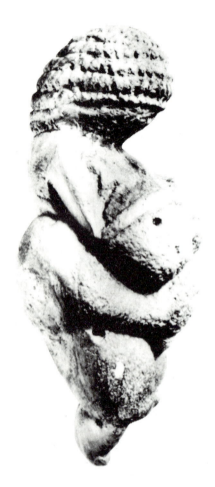

Figure 1 An early fertility symbol — emphasising the importance of fertility in society

The oldest source of information that is specifically about contraception is a papyrus from the Nile delta, thought to date from around 2000 BC, which gives information on a number of female disorders. It mentions three different methods of fertility control. The first method suggested is to sprinkle a gum-like substance derived from a tree bark exudate into the vagina to occlude the cervix. The second is to insert a paste of honey and sodium carbonate into the vagina prior to intercourse, and the third, that is recommended, is to pulverise dried crocodile dung with water to form a pessary to be inserted prior to sexual activity. Some three centuries later linen tampons were described in another medical papyrus. These were to be soaked in a mixture made of honey and a distillation of acacia shrub leaves. Interestingly, this mixture would ferment to lactic acid and a tampon soaked in this would certainly prove to be spermicidal. At the same time in other Mediterranean civilisations the insertion of a portion of sponge into the vagina was recognised as a means of preventing pregnancy. It can be appreciated therefore that the first of all forms of actual contraceptive intervention known to man was in the form of vaginal occlusion.

It is reasonable, however, to assume that the much earlier and fundamental recognition that sexual intercourse led to pregnancy gave the opportunity for fertility to be controlled by means of the man's withdrawal prior to ejaculation, and perhaps the earliest known statement of this is in Genesis 38: 7–10 where Onan 'would spill on the ground'. Coitus interruptus is not, however, artificial intervention and it is in the *Talmud* that recommendations are made for the use of what was called 'mokh'. The word is a generic term for cotton and is used particularly to mean a tampon. Similarly, in Judaic and Egyptian writings of between 500 BC and 250 AD various vegetable potions are described as being capable of making a woman 'sterile', and whilst it is doubtful that concoctions of such as Alexandrian gum (spina Aegypta), liquid alum and garden crocus acted as ovulatory suppressants, they may well have acted in an abortifacient way.

The later Greek and Roman civilisations undoubtedly understood and practised abortion as a method of fertility control. The Hippocratic book on *Diseases of Women* described a hollow lead tube which was filled with mutton fat and inserted through the cervix. The Romans made frequent use of duck quills for administering vaginal douches and for the insertion of chemical potions into the uterine cavity through the cervix. (One such instrument is on display in the museum of Haddon Hall in Derbyshire.)

The first known Greek writer to mention contraceptive methods was Aristotle, who recommended the use of olive oil to cover the surface of the cervix and the lining walls of the vagina. Olive oil does actually reduce sperm motility. Dioscorides, another Greek

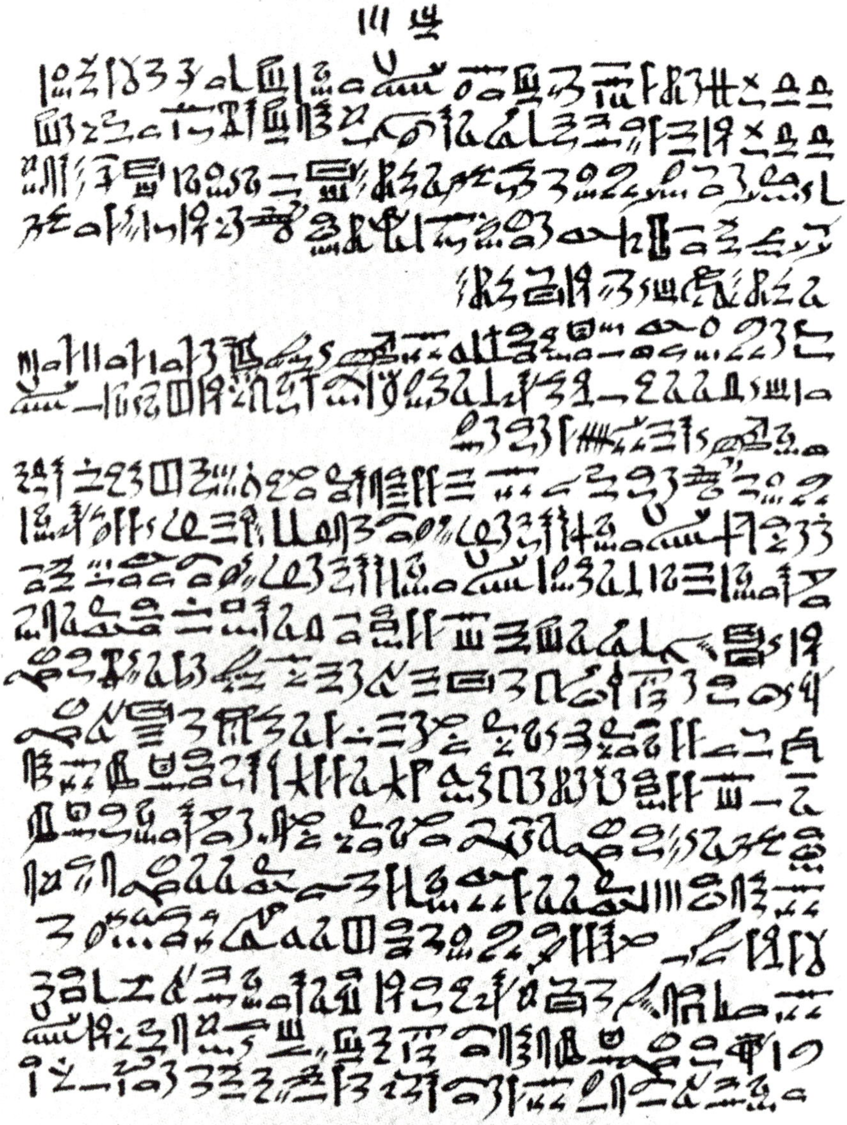

Figure 2 The Ebers Papyrus. Dated from circa 1550 BC this contains the first known reference to the use of a spermicidal chemical. (Courtesy I.P.P.F.)

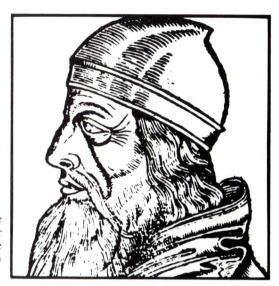

Figure 3 Aristotle — the first known Greek writer to mention contraceptive methods. (Courtesy I.P.P.F.)

physician, who wrote in the 2nd century AD, listed several herbal preparations that could be made into a pessary (Greek: 'small stone') form with honey and 'laid before conjunction to the mouth of the matrix'. Soranos a century later was more specific in his list of substances that were to be employed as vaginal barriers. He recommended oil, resin, juice of the balsam tree, myrtle essence and a woollen tampon in combination. There was little doubt that it would be effective, regardless of discomfort to the user or any difficulty in removal.

It was in Greek times that the first mention was made of any male form of intervention in the action of fertility control, although the removal of testicles, castration, had been known for millennia as a method of rendering the male (man or animal) sterile. Aetios of Amida in the 6th century recommended washing the penis in vinegar or brine, prior to intercourse. No doubt it was ineffective, though both substances are spermicidal. Four hundred years previously, however, A. Liberalis, a Roman writer, had described the problem that Minos, king of Crete, reputedly suffered from. His semen contained 'serpents', which 'injured' the women with whom he cohabited. The

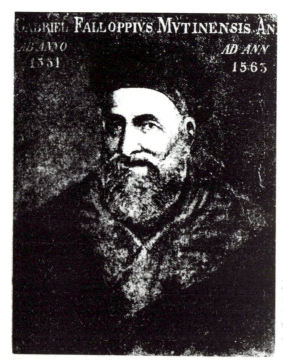

Figure 4 Gabriel Fallopius (1523–62), the first to recommend the use of a sheath to protect against disease. (Courtesy I.P.P.F.)

remedy was described as being a goat's bladder placed into the vagina of one of his concubines, into which he ejaculated. Subsequently sexual activity with his wife and queen then enabled her to conceive, for the 'serpent ridden' semen was removed. It is speculative to see this legendary story as the first ever description of a sheath, but if in those days an animal membrane encasing the penis was seen as a 'protection', it was undoubtedly possible for this method to have been employed as a contraceptive. Not until nearly a thousand years later, when Christopher Columbus had discovered the New World and brought syphilis back to the Old, did physicians take note of the sheath. Gabrielle Fallopius, the anatomist and physician, wrote in the 15th century recommending a linen sheath for the glans of the penis as a protection against disease, and from thence a multifarious variety of covers were employed. Pepys and Boswell in their *London Journals* describe the taking of 'maidens in armour'. Boswell's device was one that had to be 'dipped in the Serpentine' first, to soften it, before he rolled it on his penis 'to take his pleasure'. These were sheaths made from the caecum of a sheep, and although their widespread use in Europe for centuries was initially as a protection against venereal disease, their contraceptive effect was obviously appreciated. Casanova wrote in his book *Life* of 'that wonderful preventive against an accident which might lead to frightful repentance', and of 'the preservatives that the English have invented to put the fair sex under shelter from all fear'.

Uncertainty abounds in the literature, in modern interpretation with regard to the first descriptions of what are now called intrauterine devices (IUD). There is little doubt that for over 3000 years it was the practice of Arab camel masters, migrating with their pack-trains of animals across the continent of Africa, to insert pebbles (NB Greek 'pessary') into the uterus of their female camels to prevent unwanted pregnancy reducing the efficiency of their beast of burden. From Hippocrates to relatively modern medical writers the insertion of 'tubes' made from a variety of substances, ranging from tree bark and leather to metal, through the cervix either to theoretically enhance the prospect of conception, to secure an abortion or to correct a prolapse, was widely described. It can be assumed that since cervical and vaginal occlusion were recognised as methods of contraception since the earliest of times, it was no great step to attempt uterine cavity 'blockage'. There would be many of the occlusive pessaries recommended in early Egyptian times which would harden because of their constituents and no doubt could be inserted through a patulous cervix. Infection would remain a constant problem, however, and it is probably because of this that IUDs did not become a standard form of recommendation. In 1909 a Dr Richter of Waldenburg in Germany published a paper which described a 'thread pessary' which was for contraceptive use only, and in the 1920s, when Graefenburg developed gold and silver coiled springs, the era of the modern IUD was introduced. It had to wait until the invention of a non-toxic, non-degradable plastic in the 1940s, however, for the method to become more widely available — yet another example of technology in science advancing first before medicine could reap the benefits.

The same is true with regard to the time-honoured methods of vaginal or cervical occlusion and the sheath — it was the discovery of rubber that revolutionised their availability and use. In his treatise on gynecology published in German in 1838 Dr Friedrich Wilde described the value of taking a wax impression of a woman's cervix, then sculpturing a rubber cap to its individual shape, which she could wear 'continually to prevent a pregnancy and remove only during her menstrual period'. In 1843 the vulcanisation process for moulding and joining latex rubber was discovered and in consequence the possibility of mass producing a multiplicity of devices made from this substance emerged. From then onwards the cervical cap and sheath became ever more acceptable and convenient to use and the vaginal diaphragm developed by the anatomist Professor Mensinga in Germany in 1882 brought in a new era of increasing reliability. At the same time developments in spermicides, a principle of contraception which had been used for over five thousand years, were chemically rationalised, and the first mass production of a genuinely effective spermicidal pessary (quinine and cacao-butter combination) was undertaken in 1880 by W. J. Rendell in his London pharmaceutical factory.

At about the same time, infant milk formula began to be produced in industrial quantities; the era of artificial reproduction had begun.

Aristocrats and royalty had used wet nurses for centuries and, like Queen Victoria, had many children close together. At the end of the 19th century a decline in the duration of breastfeeding and equally important changes in patterns of suckling caused millions of women to ovulate sooner after delivery.

A century ago, therefore, scientific developments, technology and medical knowledge combined to bring to the industrial and rapidly modernising world two competing technologies. One, the increasing fertility due to artificial feeding, was neither explicitly understood nor subject to moral stricture. The other, the artificial control of fertility, was understood and ferociously resisted. In the USA Anthony Comstock persuaded Congress to make all commerce in contraception illegal. The drugs and devices developed in the 19th and early 20th centuries were more effective and acceptable but mass use was inhibited by social conservatism. Above all, research was suppressed.

John Barker, who studied spermicides in Oxford in the 1930s, was hounded from his laboratory and only rescued by Howard Florey, later famous for his work on penicillin. The US National Institute of Health, which after World War II became the world's largest funder of medical research, was expressly forbidden to work in fertility regulation until the 1960s. If social and medical priorities had been otherwise the modern woman might not have had to wait so long for the complete and easy security from the prospect of pregnancy that the pill eventually gave.

Chapter 2

Hormone Research

The history of pharmaceutical research is littered with 'accidental' discoveries. From Fleming's search in London for an antiseptic in the 1920s came the discovery in the 1940s that penicillin's growth yielded the new era of antibiotics. From Carey's search for a new insecticide in Cracow, Poland, in the 1930s came the discovery, twenty years later, that the benzodiazepines were the first generation of 'safe' tranquillisers. In hormone research, however, the physiological effects of a substance 'found' in the human body could only be surmised as the complicated biochemistry of these 'messengers' and trigger substances was and still is being slowly unravelled. In the early 1900s, for example, it was demonstrated by Haberlandt in Germany that the corpus luteum (the 'yellow' structure that appears in an ovary after a pregnancy has occurred) of one rabbit, transplanted into another, prevented the other becoming pregnant. At the same time it was not known why this occurred, but it was surmised that the corpus luteum released chemical 'messengers', i.e., hormones, that suppressed further ovulation. In 1921 Haberlandt suggested that 'extracts from ovaries' could therefore be used as oral contraceptives, but it was at least another quarter of a century before the chemical rationale could be described.

It was what is known as steroid chemistry that lagged behind the discoveries of the biologists in their theories and experiments, for they could propose an action and interaction — e.g., the corpus luteum transplant — but the chemists could not explain why, nor could they

23

by any means in the 1930s synthetically produce the substances that nature used to effect its biological control of living matter.

The term 'steroid' is derived from Greek, meaning 'like a sterol', and sterols are certain 'solid alcohols' — another chemical classification — that occur widely in plants and animals. The best known is cholesterol, which is the most abundant sterol in man and other vertebrates. All steroids share one particular kind of chemical skeleton, a series of conjugated rings (three six-membered and one five-membered) of carbon atoms to which hydrogen molecules are attached at specific points (see Figure 1). However, steroid chemistry is exceptionally complicated, because with over nineteen different points of possible attachment to the carbon atoms — each with four separate potential bonding capabilities — that form the skeleton of the molecule, there are thousands upon thousands of synthetic and naturally occurring compounds that differ only by some very minor variation in their chemical structure. Furthermore, any variation not only alters the chemical properties of the molecule but also produces dramatically different biological results. For example, based on this steroid skeleton are substances as different as all the male and female sex hormones, bile acids, blood lipids (fats), Vitamin D, the 'stress' hormones of adrenaline and cortisone and the heart stimulative constituent of digitalis. The 'only' difference between one steroid molecule and another, perhaps consisting of the introduction of an atom of oxygen at a different site, renders one substance the male sex hormone responsible, among other effects, for pubertal growth, penis enlargement, testicular production of sperm, seminal fluid secretion by the prostate gland and the cosmetic necessity of shaving (i.e., testoterone) and the other the female sex hormone responsible among other effects for breast development, uterine wall lining proliferation, cervical mucus thickening, vaginal lubrication and proneness to the psychological concomitants of premenstrual tension (i.e., progesterone).

It was the unveiling, therefore, of the mysteries of the steroid molecule, with the inevitable difficulties of testing the biological effect of what had been found when adjustments were made to that molecule, that was necessary before hormone chemistry could be even partially understood.

The structure of the steroid skeleton itself was not elucidated until 1932, when the German chemist Heinrich Wieland discovered that the most common sterol in the animal kingdom, cholesterol, possessed the specific linkage described above. Within a few years chemists in Germany, Switzerland and the USA demonstrated that testoterone, progesterone, estradiol and the adrenal hormone, cortisone, were all based on this steroid nucleus. Thus it was the European pharmaceutical companies — Ciba in Switzerland, Schering in Germany and Organon in Holland — that introduced the sex hormones into medical practice and clinical use in the late 1930s, primarily for replacement therapy in patients suffering from hormone deficiency. Chemists at these companies 'synthesised' (i.e., manufactured) testoterone (male sex hormone) and progesterone (female sex hormone) from cholesterol, by expensive and exceedingly laborious processes involving transforming the attachment of the carbon side-chain at a position on the skeleton labelled as '17' into an oxygen-containing side-chain (see Figure 1). Estradiol, the third hormone introduced into medicine at that time, could not as yet be made in this way from cholesterol and was isolated from the urine of pregnant mares, thousands of gallons of urine being necessary to produce meagre amounts of the hormone. Similarly, the conversion chemistry of cholesterol was inordinately laborious and the yield was minute. Thus all hormone treatment at that time was astronomically expensive and the substances themselves were available only in such small quantities that research into their use was inevitably limited.

In the 1940s, which historically can be seen as the decade of hormonal breakthrough, the stimulus for research was directly enhanced by the pressures of World War II. Tadeus Reichstein, a Swiss chemist, had elucidated the structure of cortisone in the late 1930s, but its synthesis from cholesterol was exceptionally difficult (since it involved at least two side-chain alterations). This 'stress' hormone, highlighted as an important aid to survival by such experiments as those conducted by Hans Selye with traumatised rats, was believed to be able to provide a potential aid to the military — the US marines in the eastern war zones and German aviators in the west — as a chemical aid to increase resistance to stress and battle fatigue. Consequently

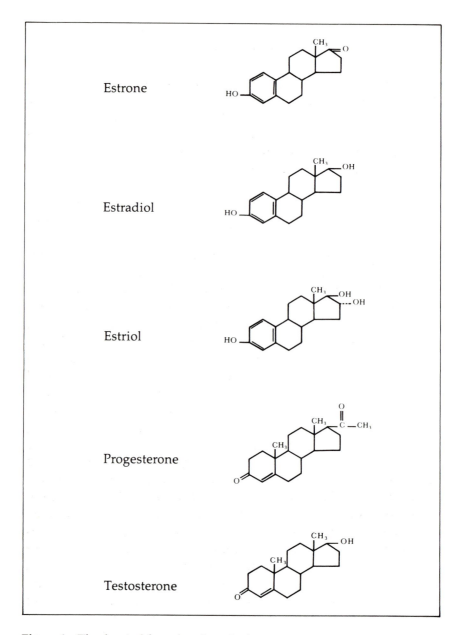

Figure 1   The chemical formulae of ovarian hormones

considerable investment went into cortisone research, notably in the major American pharmaceutical firms, Merck, Upjohn, Lederle, and Squible, and in Germany at Schering.

Lewis H. Sarrett, a young American chemist working for Merck, in 1944 accomplished the first synthesis of cortisone from cattle bile purchased from slaughterhouses. He chose this starter substance because it was the only naturally occurring steroid that already carried an oxygen atom in one of its bonds. He developed a chemical procedure for moving this atom from 'position 12' to 'position 11' and with work done by others on steroid modification added in to the procedure he produced cortisone in sufficient quantities for medical use. It was first used in 1949, on patients with rheumatoid arthritis at the Mayo Clinic, by Drs Hench and Kendall, who announced 'miraculous effects'. They were subsequently awarded the Nobel Prize for the revolutionary breakthrough in their healing work, an accident of the stimulus that came from the destruction of war.

It was a similar accidental stimulus that led to the almost simultaneous work in the hormonal field that was being undertaken alone by the American chemist Russel E. Marker, a brilliant but unorthodox professor of chemistry at Pennsylvania State University who in the early 1940s was conducting research into a group of steroids called sapogenins. These are compounds of plant origin that have this name because of the soap-like quality they show when dissolved in water. Natives of Mexico and Central America, where plants containing sapogenin occur wildly and in abundance, use them for facilitating the washing of clothes. One particular sapogenin, diosgenin, attracted Marker's attention because it had exactly the same steroid nucleus as cholesterol and only one different side-chain, and in a brilliant series of investigations he found a way to chemically degrade this side-chain and so produce a remnant steroid that was pure progesterone. 'Add-on' chemistry to the natural steroid was no longer necessary, for controlled degradation was much simpler, but the consequences of Marker's research were yet to be realised by everyone except Marker himself. He discovered diosgenin was particularly abundant in certain types of Mexican yam and he urged the pharmaceutical company Parke-Davis which was supporting his university research to capitalise on his discovery. They were not interested, so Marker gave up his academic appointment, went to Mexico and on his own arranged for the collection from the countryside around Vera Cruz of over ten tons of the yam species known as 'cabaza de negro' (black-headed yam). He rented a laboratory in Mexico City, where he supervised the extraction of the syrupy substance diosgenin. Returning to the States he used the industrial laboratory of a friend to purify the extract into more than three kilograms of the human sex hormone progesterone, which at that time was worth more than US $80 a gram. Having demonstrated alone that progesterone could easily be prepared in prodigious quantities, and relatively inexpensively in comparison with any other known procedure, Marker decided to establish a production facility in Mexico, nearer the source of the naturally occurring yam. Looking through the telephone directory under the heading 'Laboratory', he noticed the name 'Laboratorios Hormona'. Contacting the owners, Drs Somlo and Lehmann, Marker demonstrated his discovery and forming a new company, Syntex (the name derived from 'synthesis' and 'Mexico'), in which he retained a 40% share, on 21 January 1944, he founded the first pharmaceutical company with the capability of relatively cheap mass production of a human sex hormone.

Progesterone had been released onto the international market for pharmaceutical research and medical use, with widespread availability in large quantities. But it was still to be twenty years before the pill was born.

Chapter 3

The First Use of Hormonal Contraception ?

The physiologist Ludwig Haberlandt who had explored the possibility of the use of ovarian extracts in his animal experiments had written, in 1931: '. . . of all methods available, hormonal sterilization based on biological principles, if it can be applied unobjectionably in the human, is an ideal method for practical medicine and its future task of birth control.'

Haberlandt's vision was unique and the work that was done in sex hormones in the following decades was for everything *except* contraception. Attempts were made to extract ovarian hormones from such a variety of sources as the amniotic fluid of cows in Germany, pregnant mares' urine in Switzerland and the USA, and the sweet potato in Japan. In 1936 in Holland less than 25 mg of estradiol was derived from four tons of sows' ovaries. Plainly, the pathetic and expensive yield, until Russell Marker perfected his extraction process of such rich sources as the Mexican yam, defeated any attempts at research into widespread use of the hormonal substances that were involved in ovulation or fertility control. By 1950, however, through Marker's work steroid hormones became available at one hundredth of the price they had cost a decade previously.

Carl Djerassi, another leading pioneer in hormone chemistry, was in 1949 a 25-year-old post-graduate working in New Jersey at the American branch of the Swiss pharmacautical firm Ciba. His PhD thesis from the University of Wisconsin was on the chemical conversion of the male sex hormone testoterone into the female sex hormone estradiol. Because of this he received an invitation to join

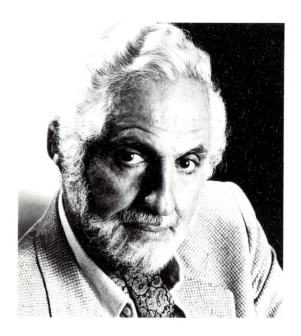

Figure 1 Carl Djerassi

the workers at Syntex in Mexico City, who had been temporarily devastated by Marker's abrupt departure and desertion of chemistry. He joined George Rosenkrantz, by then Vice-President of Syntex (a Hungarian who had emigrated from Switzerland to Cuba before being recruited by Syntex), who had also done his PhD in steroid chemistry and who, because of his knowledge of sapogenin research, had developed a technique for commercially synthesising testoterone (male sex hormone), also from the prized Mexican yam. Djerassi, exploring all these synthesis possibilit:es, then went on at Syntex to produce cortisone, both from Marker's diosgenin (yam-derived) and from another sapogenin which was available from the waste products of Mexican sisal (jute) production. This manufacturing process of steroid hormones from plant raw material, rather than from the much more expensive and difficult animal sources, made Syntex the leading supplier of steroids to the rest of the world's pharmaceutical industry.

Clinically, the hormone progesterone was at that time being used in trials to treat various menstrual disorders, including painful periods,

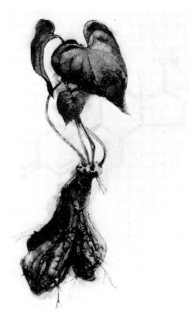

Figure 2 The Mexican yam that Dr Marker used to obtain progesterone

to prevent miscarriage and in one centre to treat cancer of the cervix. Over a dozen years earlier, however, Hans H. Inhoffen and his colleagues in the research laboratories at Schering had been experimenting with chemical alterations of the molecules of estradiol and testoterone and had found that once artificially changed (by acetylene introduced at position 17) the molecule of the male hormone, testoterone, acted clinically, yet surprisingly, as a female sex hormone — progesterone. Djerassi and his colleagues in 1951 followed on with this work to further alter the hormonal molecules and discovered that if progesterone had both its '17' group and its '19' group of bonded atoms changed, then a substance termed '19-norprogesterone' and subsequently 'norethisterone' could be made. Later clinical assessment of this new hormonal substance demonstrated that it was infinitely far more active as a progestational hormone, taken by mouth, than any other steroid known at the time. Suddenly synthesised steroids that were chemically tailored for high effectiveness became available. But Haberlandt had been forgotten and every possible use, except

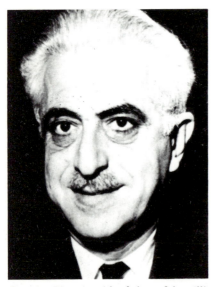

Gregory Pincus — 'the father of the pill'

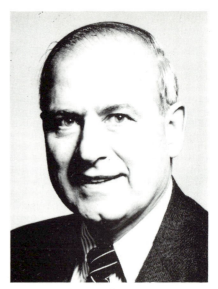

Ramon Garcia

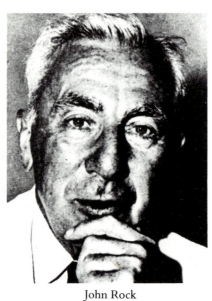

John Rock

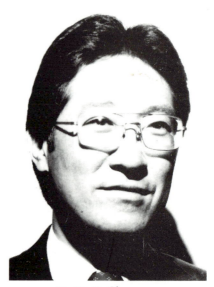

Dr M. C. Chang

Figure 3

contraception, was explored. 'Not in our wildest dreams did we imagine that eventually this substance would become the active progestational ingredient of over 50% of currently used oral contraceptives', wrote Carl Djerassi, looking back in 1979 on the impact of their discovery eighteen years earlier.

A few weeks after synthesising this substance, norethisterone (called norethindrone in the USA), Syntex sent it to various endocrinologists and clinicians for assessment: Roy Hertz at the National Cancer Institute, Gregory Pincus at the Worcester Foundation, Robert Greenblatt in Georgia and Edward Tyler in Los Angeles. In November 1954 Edward Tyler of the Los Angeles Planned Parenthood Centre presented the first clinical results of the use of norethisterone in the treatment of menstrual disorders and fertility problems.

Meanwhile, in August 1953 Frank D. Colton of Searle had filed a patent for the synthesis of a substance very closely related to norethisterone (norethynodrel, which differed only by the location of the double bond between positions '5' and '10', rather than '4' and '5', but which on exposure to weak hydrochloric acid, as in the human stomach, actually became largely norethisterone).

Thus it was that in 1953–4 two similar agents exerting an intense progesterone effect in small doses when taken by mouth became available for use by clinicians in their treatment of human beings and their assessment of hormonal effect, the one from Syntex and the other from Searle.

Gregory Pincus, a biologist of the Worcester Foundation, Massachusetts, M. C. Chang, a collaborator, and John Rock, a clinician at Harvard, were also interested in the chemical achievement of ovulatory inhibition and found that these products were the two most active steroids in that respect. Nine years earlier Albright, at Harvard, had foreseen a potential use for orally active steroids beyond the confines of gynecological treatment and had speculated: 'Since preventing ovulation prevents pregnancy, one could employ the same principles in birth control as preventing dysmenorrhea (painful periods).' Nevertheless, it was perhaps only due to the drive of the American social 'worker' for women's 'rights', Margaret Sanger, and the philanthropy of Mrs Page McCormick from the family that owned International

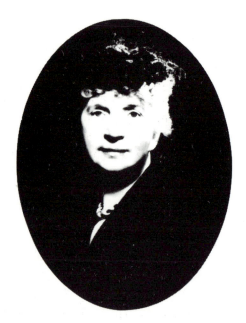

Figure 4 Margaret Sanger (1883–1966), an early campaigner for better information about birth control. (Courtesy I.P.P.F.)

Harvester that the first oral contraceptive was actually developed with rapidity from then onwards, for a grant of US $115 000 was given in 1954 to Pincus, Chang and the Catholic obstetrician, Rock, to undertake animal and human research into effective 'hormonal birth control'. Even allowing for inflation it was a small sum of money to set off a drug revolution, and later many times that sum was to be spent on studying the effects of the birth control pills.

It was then that an interesting diversion in the commercial development of the first form of the pill took place, with religious conviction, economic politics, and the murky waters of competition over patent rights all involved.

Pincus, a consultant for Searle, understandably picked the Searle compound (patented in 1954, some eighteen months after Djerassi and his colleagues at Syntex had released the first active form of norethisterone) for use in his biological and the clinical studies. It was first tried on a small group of human volunteers in Boston. However, at this time contraception was still illegal in Massachusetts, under the 19th century laws promoted by Comstock. The US Supreme Court was to strike down these laws only in 1967 in the celebrated case of

Griswood versus Connecticut. Margaret Sanger had been imprisoned under Comstock laws and then in the 1930s family planning pioneers, by involving physicians, had won a limited right to give advice on grounds of health, but clearly Massachusetts was not an ideal place to try a fundamentally new contraceptive. The need for a large clinical trial was obvious; this was conducted in Puerto Rico and demonstrated that the ovulation inhibition properties of norethisterone 'could be employed for contraceptive purposes as well as for menstrual regulation'. The results were published in the *Science Journal* in 1956 under the euphemistic title of 'Effects of certain 19-norsteroids on the normal human menstrual cycle' by the authors Rock, Pincus and Garcia (a young gynecologist who was the Puerto Rican clinical collaborator and who also worked with Edris Rice-Wray, the first female physician involved in testing the pill).

Technically, the substance used in this very first trial was only almost accidentally effective. It was Searle's particular form of synthetic progesterone and Pincus, who had actually started out with John Rock, the clinician of Boston, to investigate the feasibility of its use to improve fertility, was unaware that it actually contained an estrogen-like component, later to be defined as mestranol. Rock was a Catholic and the rationale for treating his patients in Boston with the new synthetic hormones to inhibit ovulation was in the hope that when the course of treatment was stopped the ovaries would 'rebound' in their reaction to artificial suppression by producing more follicles, thus enhancing the woman's fertility and enabling her to conceive. There was some evidence of this effect, so the Catholic gynecologist, whose main interest was in fertility stimulation, accidentally became involved in the development of the world's first effective form of oral contraception.

These two accidents, for such they were, and it is only with hindsight that their irony can be appreciated, were accompanied by a third, one which left several major pharmaceutical firms way behind their competitors in this developing field.

It must be recalled that it was Djerassi and colleagues at Syntex who had produced and patented the first synthetic norethisterone, some eighteen months before Colton at Searle had produced his version.

Syntex had no marketing organisation for its pharmaceutical products and so needed to collaborate with another company. Parke-Davis was chosen, since it was notably behind in the steroid field, and it needed a product for the growing area of treatment of 'menstrual disorders and certain conditions of infertility'. Syntex therefore provided Parke-Davis with all the laboratory and preliminary clinical data accumulated so far, as well as with additional results from animal studies (done on monkeys), in an exclusive agreement of licence in 1956. Similarly an option was on offer from Syntex to Charles Pfizer and Company, now part of the multi-national Cynamid. In both cases concern about potential Catholic reaction to the production of a contraceptive agent led to further progress being halted. In one it was the personal and religious-based stance of the company's president, and in the other it was the fear of the loss of sales of its anti-seasickness pills from Catholic customers, that resulted in the decisions not to proceed.

Thus, with these complexities all playing their part, it was not the Syntex form of norethisterone that was used when the large-scale human trial of oral contraception was started in Rio Piedras, Puerto Rico, but Searle's version. Pincus, described since as a 'masterful scientific entrepreneur', had utilised the forces of his own 'eloquence and persuasion' to ensure that Searle manufactured their product as an oral contraceptive, and they obtained approval for its licence in 1959, two years after its initial approval as a 'menstrual regulator'. Recognising the political and religious ramifications of the time, Egon Diczfalusy, leader of the WHO Task Force on Contraceptive Development, wrote in 1979: 'Full credit should be given to the Searle Company for their sang-froid, vision and courage in marketing the first oral contraceptive preparation in 1959 in a hostile atmosphere controlled by restrictive and conservative societal forces influenced by traditionalism, strong taboos (and still popular) belief that techno-logical progress can be stopped by ideological forces and political determination. This was a period in history when several drug houses declared that it was and always would be incompatible with their ethical principles to manufacture fertility regulating agents.'

Meanwhile, however, although the initial substance from Searle, norethynodrel, had proved successful and acceptable to the women of Puerto Rico, when it came to the scaling up of its synthesis 'impurities' were removed. The use of the purer progesterone then led to serious problems that included not only severe menstrual irregularities and unacceptable breakthrough bleeding, but also pregnancies. Urgent investigation of the difference showed that the original product actually contained just over 1% of an estrogen type of chemical substance, called mestranol. This was therefore put back in the preparation by Searle in a standardised level of 1.5% and the progestogen-estrogen pill was born. The final accident in the chapter of discoveries had occurred and the birth of the 'birth control' pill had become history. Seven years had passed since Djerassi and his colleagues had synthesised the orally active progesterone, norethisterone, before the first commercially available contraceptive pill, Enavid, became available on prescription to women in the United States. Not only were contraceptives *de jure* illegal but abortion was unthinkable. As a consequence women were seriously overdosed with the first oral contraceptives. In most drug development the dose is raised until the desired therapeutic effect is achieved. In the case of the pill the reverse was true and the dose was cautiously lowered over the first twenty years of use. The dose in some of the early pills was up to a hundred times that which is used today. This byway of history resulted in the early pill being associated with an unnecessarily high rate of side-effects and in the death of some women who otherwise would have lived. Epidemiology — which always reads yesterday's experiences — saw a more dangerous drug than was necessary.

The next decades, therefore, were involved not in a race to discover new products but in evaluation and modification of what had already been achieved. The 'giant step' for women and human society had been taken in Puerto Rico in 1955.

Chapter 4

The Impact of Social Changes
due to the Pill

In the 1950s and early 1960s contraception was not a feature of the average physician's or family doctor's practice; there were probably few gynecologists even who saw it as part of their work. The attitude of the medical profession to what was jokingly called the 'rubber goods trade' was one of distinct disdain that had changed little in the previous twenty-five years or more. In 1923, for example, reflecting what was perhaps a standard opinion, the editor of the *Practitioner* had written: 'The subject of birth control is not taught in the medical schools and in the case of schools for male students it is safe to predict that it never will be: for women are more practical and less hypocritical than most men.' In 1930 the students at Newcastle University Medical School invited the doctor from the local birth control clinic to address the Students Medical Society. When the authorities learnt of this they warned the students' committee that anyone attending 'would run the risk of failure in the final examinations'. The meeting was cancelled. In 1950, when the Deans of the twenty-four medical schools in the UK were asked about the provision of birth control instruction for qualifying doctors in their schools, in a survey conducted by the Federation of Medical Women, it was found that it was provided at only four of them. By 1960 it had become a 'voluntary' subject for medical students in medical school, which meant in most cases an evening visit to a Family Planning Clinic in the local town, as part of the Public Health curriculum. The visit was not compulsory, no formal instruction was given, 'and embarrassment was equal on both the part of the

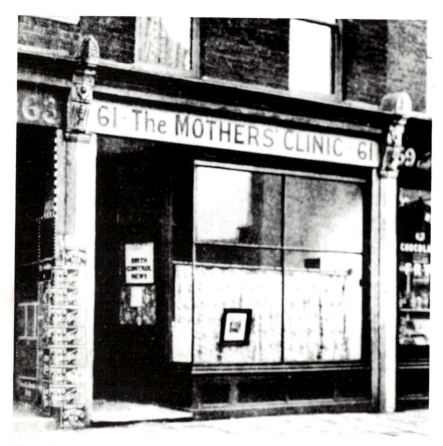

Figure 1 One of the first Family Clinics to be established — Marie Stope's clinic in the Holloway district of London, established in 1921. (Courtesy I.P.P.F.)

student seeing a tray of strange shaped rubber caps on display and the women who were attending the clinic sitting in queues with their stockings rolled down waiting their turn to lie, in lithotomy position, on the one couch behind the rather dirty curtain'.

At that stage, in the early 1960s, the Family Planning Clinics would give appointments only to married women or those 'with a printed invitation to their forthcoming wedding'. Qualified doctors and students in training received virtually no instruction at all in contraception, and abortion was illegal (in the UK until 1972). Yet the first oral contraceptive, Enavid, suddenly became available on a 'private' prescription from general practitioners (it could not initially be prescribed under the terms of the National Health Service), who were thus able to charge a small fee for its provision. In January 1962 (a year after its licence was granted in the USA) Searle's Enavid started to be taken by women in the UK. Within five years the GPs' 'pocket money' from this source was rising considerably as women in their tens of thousands were asking for the prescriptions.

Many doctors resisted their patients' requests, some for religious and some for their own 'aesthetic' reasons, so local authorities and clinics started to provide a free service, selling supplies of the pill at discount prices to their clients. By the 1970s the situation was regularised in the so-called 'Doctors' Charter' negotiated with the Department of Health by the Doctors' Salaries Review Body, whereby a special item of service fee was provided to GPs for each patient who registered with them for contraceptive services. In return the GP was obliged to follow the recommendations of the *Handbook of Contraceptive Practice* issued by the Standing Medical Advisory Committee with regard to the assessment of patients, their screening and surveillance. Cynically it might be said that it was either because of the fees involved or because of the almost overwhelming demand for the provision of service (i.e., to get the pill) from their women patients that so many GPs then undertook to become involved in contraception. Certainly, by 1976 an enquiry among British GPs found that 93% 'advised individuals on contraceptive matters', although only just over 30% of them had received any training whatsoever on the subject in their undergraduate or post-graduate years. The medical profession had been dragged willy-nilly into a field of care they knew little about and that previously they had viewed with remarkable disdain.

The 'early' pills marketed in the UK — Enavid by Searle, and soon afterwards Ortho-Novum from Ortho Pharmaceuticals and then Anovlar from Schering — contained what is now realised to have been a massive overdosage of hormone. (The reduction in hormone content subsequently, without any loss of contraceptive security, has been a hundred-fold.) In consequence, and not surprisingly, the incidence of side-effects in the women who took them was considerable. Breast tenderness, migraine, weight increase, depression of libido, menstrual suppression on ceasing the medication regime and a host of other unwanted effects were experienced. Nevertheless, to a generation of women who had never previously known any form of totally reliable contraception at all, the pill was a positive boon. There were certainly few 'drop outs' in the early years, despite the side-effects, although some cautious doctors recommended, without any scientific evidence at that stage for doing so, that their patients on the pill should have 'a rest from taking it' periodically. Perhaps because the idea grew that it worked by mimicking pregnancy, the usual suggestion was to take it for nine months consecutively and then to come 'off it' for three. This myth still continues in some minds even today. (It was in fact also an echo of the earliest of all 'suggestions' in the licensing considerations of the FDA in the United States in 1959, when the oral contraceptive norethisterone was being assessed based on the evidence of a study of only 132 women.)

Nevertheless, the ever-increasing use of the pill by sexually active women and the restriction on access to it (by contrast to all other then available forms of contraception, which could be bought by mail order, purchased from chemists, 'surgical stores' or even hairdressers) as being only through the medical profession brought about two quite dramatic changes in public attitudes, that have continued ever since.

Firstly, there was a social revolution in sexual attitudes — no other word can describe the change. Oral contraception literally 'released' men and women from the consequence of sexual intercourse being pregnancy, and its name 'the pill' became part of contemporary language as having only one particular meaning. A morality of behaviour, going back tens of thousands of years through the history of human society, had been based on fear — the fear that sex led to pregnancy. Suddenly these two consecutive circumstances were separated. As a result not only attitudes but also behaviour changed. The media termed those early years of pill availability the 'Swinging Sixties', authorities (and parents) expressed their fears that the pill 'made young women have sex', there were claims that 'it threatened the stability of marriage', and rearguard actions on behalf of older generations and religious groups were fought long and hard.

The second dramatic change came about as a result of the medical profession's involvement in the provision of contraception. Since doctors are almost invariably linked with illness, contraception involving the use of the pill inevitably became an 'illness-associated' routine. To 'go on' the pill a woman 'had to submit' to a form of physical check-up, probably involving a vaginal examination (currently perhaps a cervical cytology test), breast examination and other routine assessments. For repeat prescriptions the ritual of a 'medical examination' was continued; indeed it is part of the current requirements of the *Handbook of Contraceptive Practice*. In the interests of women's health the need for this cannot be gainsaid, and in fact they are now (the group of the female population who are using contraceptives that involve medical 'intervention', i.e., diaphragm, IUD, and pill) the only sector of the population in the UK with a National Health Service provision and fee payment arrangement that ensure they have a periodic health check-up. A consequence of this will inevitably be better health expectancy due to the earlier diagnosis of disorder, disease and degenerative illness. Nevertheless, it has meant that a loss of virginity for a young woman has to be 'admitted' to a third party, the doctor who is consulted for contraceptive advice; that 'safe' sexual activity, free from the fear of pregnancy for any woman of reproductive age, involves consulting doctors; and that doctors hold an authoritative position over something that to the woman is (or was) essentially private and personal. The subtleties of all this mean that illness, doctors, health and contraception are all inseparably linked, a situation that only the pill has 'achieved', as a mixed blessing, in the last two decades.

Chapter 5

The 'Image' of the Pill
— a Remarkable Social Change

F. Riphagen

Now, thirty years after its discovery, the oral contraceptive is the most widely employed form of modern fertility control, being used by more than sixty million women of fertile age world-wide, about equally divided between developing and developed countries (and an equally large number have used it in the past).

Thirty years of history have also witnessed constant progress in the pharmaceutical development of the preparations used, changes in the formulation having been brought about by quite unique long-term studies of the pill and its effects, such as those done by the Royal College of General Practitioners of the UK, the Family Planning Association, and the Centers for Disease Control of the United States.

At the same time, and by no coincidence, there has been a social evolution in Western developed countries with regard to sexual 'morality' and behaviour. The development of the pill undoubtedly opened the door to further separation of sexuality and procreation. Sexual liberty became a theme of the sixties and the seventies, when moral values changed and secularisation advanced. However, it is important to note that sexual habits, as measured for example by registered cases of sexually transmitted disease, rose before the wide-spread availability of oral contraceptives in the 1960s.

Meanwhile, medical science began to concentrate on the prevention of serious diseases, such as cardio-vascular disease and cancer. Health politicians realised that dramatic improvements in health care as seen in the battle against infectious diseases, malnutrition and unhygienic living conditions belonged to the past. Health education was introduced as the new tool to help people to improve their life-style: a reduction in smoking, less drinking and eating and more physical exercise were supposed to add longevity for everyone. At the same time, social services became increasingly important and in many countries the 'Welfare State' appeared, supposed to take care of all the needs, present and future, of its people.

The older and newer means of mass-communication, the news-papers, magazines and television, played and still play an important role in the distribution of the modern health information and changes in social policy. Today, no newspaper, magazine or television channel can be found without its own medical column or programme. In consequence, attitudes and perceptions have changed, often subtly, among populations who nowadays gain medical information not only from their doctors but also from the media. A new era of influence and expectations has therefore emerged.

The ever-increasing popularity of the pill has to be set into the context of this evolution that has taken place in Western developed countries. Oral contraception can be regarded as one of the hallmarks of social and medical development, and as regards the present situation it has been perhaps aptly described by Kay, who labelled it 'the happiness pill'[1]. Nevertheless, in recent decades the public view has swung considerably.

In 1984 and 1985 the International Health Foundation conducted surveys of knowledge, attitudes and the practices of contraception in five West European countries: Italy, France, Great Britain, Spain and the Federal Republic of Germany. These studies included some 8400 women between 15 and 45 years of age. The questionnaire assessed general perceptions of all methods of contraception and also included a detailed section on the possible advantages and disadvantages of the pill[2-6]. Running parallel with the European surveys was a joint opinion poll conducted by Family Health International and the International Health Foundation in thirteen countries world-wide, including Spain and the Federal Republic of Germany[7]. This opinion poll contained a limited number of questions that were similar to those included in the poll conducted in the United States by Gallup, at the request of the American College of Obstetricians and Gynecologists in 1985[8].

GENERAL PERCEPTIONS

Users and potential users nowadays 'judge' methods of contraception, including their reliability, on both moral and religious acceptability, interference with sex life, and safety for health. The results of the surveys in the five West European countries are given in Figures 1–4 in a schematic way. Scales go from positive (left), doubt (middle), to negative (right). These three zones are well defined. Barrier methods are those of the condom, the diaphragm and spermicides together, the latter two, however, nowhere reaching a user rate of 1% each.

Natural methods represent rhythm and withdrawal, which are here grouped together for clarity.

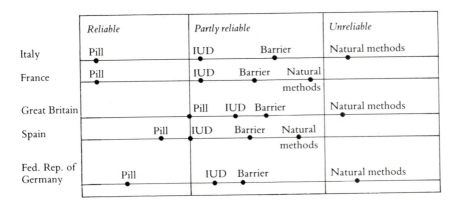

Figure 1   Perceived reliability of contraceptive methods

In comparison with the other methods, the pill is considered to be reliable (Figure 1), with only Great Britain in the 'doubt' zone but very close to the cutting off point.

Figure 2, showing moral and religious acceptability, indicates that motives of this nature do not appear to be discriminating as all methods are considered acceptable in all five countries.

In the case of Spain and Italy, one must remember that in these two countries surgical sterilisation for contraceptive reasons is very uncommon.

Acceptable
Partly acceptable
Unacceptable
Italy
Pill IUD Natural
Barrier methods
Steril.
France
Pill IUD Nat.
Barrier Steril.
Great Britain
Barrier Steril.
Nat. IUD
Pill
Spain
Pill IUD Nat.
Barrier
Steril.
Fed. Rep. of Germany
Pill IUD Nat.
Barrier Steril.

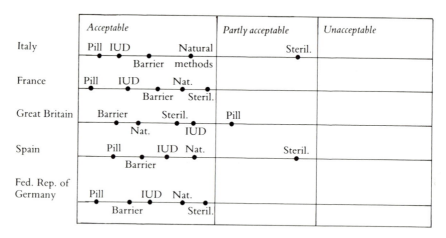

Figure 2 Perceived moral and religious acceptability

Interference by contraceptive methods in sex life, as shown in Figure 3 for a few relevant methods, is, however, perceived differently. In all five countries the pill obtains good marks and is not considered to interfere with sex life.

Finally, safety for health, shown for some relevant methods, is pre-

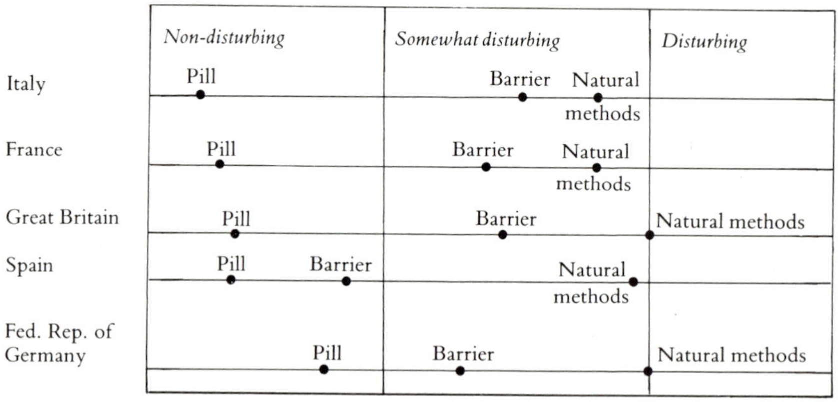

Non-disturbing
Somewhat disturbing
Disturbing
Italy
Pill
Barrier Natural methods
France
Pill
Barrier Natural methods
Great Britain
Pill
Barrier
Natural methods
Spain
Pill Barrier
Natural methods
Fed. Rep. of Germany
Pill
Barrier
Natural methods

Figure 3 Perceived disturbance of sex life, by contraceptive methods

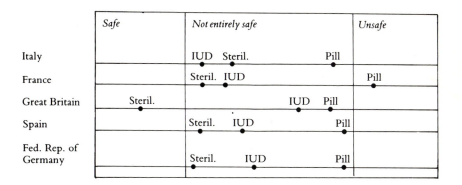

	Safe	Not entirely safe			Unsafe
Italy		IUD Steril.		Pill	
France		Steril. IUD			Pill
Great Britain	Steril.		IUD Pill		
Spain		Steril. IUD		Pill	
Fed. Rep. of Germany		Steril. IUD		Pill	

Figure 4 Perceived safety for health of some contraceptive methods

sented in Figure 4. Clearly, there is much doubt about the safety of the pill, and in the case of France it is even considered 'unsafe'.

These overall perceptions of contraceptive methods are remarkably similar in the different countries, notwithstanding the considerable differences in usage rates. Pill use, for instance, varies greatly from Italy (5%) and Spain (13%) to France (26%), West Germany (30%) and Great Britain (31%). Evidently, public opinion does not stop at national borders. A second observation is that, from a medical point of view, the results seem to correspond well with present knowledge about reliability, moral and religious acceptability and the 'disturbance of sex life' factor of these contraceptive methods.

The supposed danger to users' health, however, appears to be overestimated in all the countries studied. The ubiquitous association of the pill and to a smaller degree of the IUD with disease is thus distinctly out of proportion to the medical eye.

Clearly, the pill is nowadays the most widely known method of contraception (which was also shown in this five-country study by the fact that its use was greatly overestimated by the women questioned). In the Federal Republic of Germany, for instance, the respondents thought that 82% of the women in the country used the pill, while only 30% in fact used it. Similar differences were found in the other four countries.

The association of oral contraceptives with a danger to health is the more important because 'health motives' have turned out to be by far the most important reason initiating a change of contraceptive method. In the near future, therefore, women in Great Britain, West Germany and France will, it can be assumed, attach even more importance to the 'health issue', while reliability, the primary feature of contraceptive methods for many years, will presumably become less important in these countries.

The overall image of contraceptive methods shows nowadays, thirty years after its discovery, that quite clearly oral contraceptives are considered reliable, acceptable and beneficial for sex life, but 'unhealthy' — a dramatic change in view.

THE SPECIFIC IMAGE OF THE PILL

The perceived advantages and disadvantages of the oral contraceptive have been analysed to obtain a more detailed insight into what has led women to form their point of view of the pill. They fall into short-term, reversible side-effects, long-term and serious disease, disadvantages of a non-medical nature and advantages of varying nature.

Reversible side-effects

Weight gain was attributed to the pill by women in all five countries (70–85% were either sure or thought it possible that the pill makes one gain weight).

Headache came in second place here, especially in Great Britain and West Germany (65 and 68%), but to a lesser degree in the other three countries (36 to 39%).

Painful tension of the breasts was noticed especially in West Germany (58%), Italy (51%) and Great Britain (47%), but less often in Spain and France.

Nervousness was quite frequently associated with the oral contraceptive (Great Britain 30%, West Germany 47%, and France 60%).

Depressive moods was a response in West Germany (54%) and Great Britain (55%), while in the other three coutries around 30% reported these.

Vaginal infection was also associated with use of oral contraceptives (35% in Great Britain, and between 14 and 26% in the other countries).

Irregular bleeding (spotting) was most often thought to be linked to the use of the pill in West Germany (58%), while in other countries between 18 and 36% of pill-users made the association.

These results concerning reversible side-effects are correlated to current or past experience with the pill, since the number of women in the surveys who stated 'no idea' were higher in Spain and Italy, where current and past use is lower than in the other three countries.

Past and current users together constitute around 50% of the studied groups in Germany and France, considerably more in Great Britain (85%), but only 33 and 39% in Italy and Spain.

Some of these differences are probably due to the fact that most women today use modern low-dose pills, containing less estrogen and sometimes newer progestogen compounds. Furthermore, pharmacological developments have enabled doctors to practise individual prescribing, since they have gathered more experience themselves and have more choice in formulations. Non-users in these study samples therefore seem to be more responsible for the 'negativism' concerning side-effects. In other words, they have not been adequately informed of the improvements in oral contraception over the last twenty-five years.

Other supposed disadvantages

The *obligation to take a pill every day* at least for twenty-one days in a row and for a long period of time, when one is healthy, has been supposed to 'wear out' users' motivation. Actual experience of current users is apparently less troublesome everywhere with the exception of France, where a large proportion of current users (59%) indicate that this is indeed a problem.

A *lowered libido* associated with use of the pill was correlated most in West Germany (40%), while in the other countries it affected only around 20%.

Financial cost was not considered to be a disadvantage of oral contraceptives in any of the five countries studied.

Long-term irreversible side-effects

In this category three aspects have been assessed with regard to the 'public view': infertility after long duration of use, a higher risk of malignant disease (unspecified) and cardio-vascular disease. These three conditions were selected because it was felt that they have received a lot of attention and publicity over the years.

Infertility after long duration of pill use was a strong association in West Germany (71%) and Great Britain (60%). France followed with 46% and Italy and Spain were behind with 32 and 25% respectively. Though all the scientific evidence has been much more reassuring, many women still think that oral contraception 'makes them sterile'[9].

Increased cancer risk was supposed to be associated with oral contraceptive use by 69% of the questioned women in Great Britain. (France, Italy and West Germany 45%, Spain 30%.)

As in the other opinion views, the results here are disproportionally high and out of touch with current scientific evidence[10]. The present state of affairs regarding breast cancer is relatively reassuring, but due to the numerous contradictory publications in medical journals and subsequently in the newspapers women cannot be blamed for being confused and therefore suspicious[11-14].

A higher risk of cardio-vascular disease has hung on in the minds of many women in Great Britain (59%) and France (52%), and in the other three countries around 40% held the association.

Both associations shown by the CSM report (thrombo-embolism) and the Royal College of General Practitioners Study (smoking, age over 35 and cardio-vascular disease) have been followed by pharmacological developments and considerable improvements in the pill's formulation[12, 13]. Estrogen doses were lowered and thrombo-embolism incidence went down, and progestogen doses were lowered too, or replaced by newer non-androgenic substances which do not affect the relevant blood lipid spectrum.

The 'medical news' is therefore good, but apparently both pill-users and non-users alike still live in the past to a considerable degree.

Advantages

The responses here in the surveys consisted mainly of immediately noticeable features of a practical nature.

Cycle regularity was a widespread feature (from 62% for Italy to 94% in West Germany).

The same was observed for the improvement of dysmenorrhea, where percentages from 46% for Italy to 86% for West Germany were found. Having less painful periods appears to be a true benefit, which it is of course, and a considerable one if we consider the amount of accumulated sick leave caused by dysmenorrhea.

The *ease of use* was overwhelmingly recognised, and here the scores were 80% and higher.

More general advantages such as *absence of disturbance of sex life* and *reliability* were already found to be widely recognised.

As to the set of advantages involved, the recorded opinions of the studied women seem well in correspondence with reality.

All this confirms and explains the general perception that the studied women have of oral contraceptives: reliable, acceptable, easy to use, with very clear advantages, but bad for one's health. Reversible side-effects are overestimated, especially when the estimates of users and non-users are compared. The most serious misconceptions among users and non-users alike concern serious, irreversible and long-term effects.

SOURCES OF INFORMATION

In each of the five countries studied, about 50% of the women indicated that they obtained important information on contraception and the method currently used from sources such as magazines and newspapers, television, friends and relatives, in short non-professional sources. Professional sources took care of the other 50%.

In the case of the bad image of the pill, there has evidently been a problem of communication leading to misinformation of the public, both men and women. It is very unlikely that a single, one-way mechanism is at work here, consisting of telling only wrong things to people who in turn believe all they are told. Undoubtedly, there are some members of the medical and family planning disciplines who omit to relay sufficient information to their patients. Equally the way some newspapers and magazines sometimes carry incomplete and inexact stories about the pill has certainly led to misunderstanding. However, it would be wrong to point the accusing finger at either the media or the medical profession, because the responsibility for accurate and suitable information is a joint one.

The news

The day-to-day experience of doctors prescribing oral contraceptives over the last twenty-five years has brought to light a number of relatively harmless side-effects, such as, for instance, headache and weight gain. It has also led to a set of well defined contra-indications for oral contraceptives, for instance, hypertension, and liver disease. A much wider dimension, however, has been added by large-scale epidemiological studies. The publication of a report for the Committee for the Safety of Medicines in 1970, relating a higher incidence of thrombo-embolic disease in pill-users to the estrogen compounds in the combined pills, was the first example[15].

The 'Oral Contraceptives and Health' study group of the Royal College of General Practitioners' Manchester Research Unit followed up with several publications of results of its large prospective study[16,17].

Other examples are studies by the Oxford Family Planning Association and the Center for Disease Control Studies in the USA[18–20]. A great number of possible associations between oral contraceptives and various diseases and conditions have been investigated.

The public received its information about the health effects of the pill in the first place out of these epidemiological studies not through their physician and from the same sources, but via various means of mass communication. Other sources are manufacturers' package inserts and informal circuits, i.e., gossip.

The prescribing physician and epidemiology

Epidemiologists are very often the first to point out the methodological weaknesses of their own work and realise the difficulties in performing large long-term studies. They are also very concerned to describe their results as 'positive or negative associations' instead of causal relationships. The fact that different studies sometimes produce different results is not uncommon in epidemiological research. In the case of the pill, the number of factors to be taken into account, including duration of use, age at first use, parity and age at first pregnancy, to name a few, is disappointingly great.

The prescribing doctor depends on the results of these studies to inform his patients. In the case of the pill this is not easy, because of the conflicting, inconclusive nature of some of the relevant material and the sometimes small but not insignificant size of the obtained results, especially when they concern rare diseases, such as liver cancer, for example. Not every pill-prescribing doctor is entirely familiar with epidemiology, but, even so, he has to point out this kind of information relating to use, during consultations.

A further problem is that doctors deal with individual patients who might not find it easy to make their decisions with the aid of statistics, even when they are not confused. In the best of cases, the doctor might present his patients with a complete and accurate balance of benefits and risks of oral contraceptives, indicating what might and might not happen to 10 000 women who take the pill, but even so an individual woman will find it hard to appreciate her own 'statistical risk'. Thus professional communication has its hazards. In the last analysis, perhaps what the woman really wants to know is 'Doctor, would you or your wife use the pill?'

The media and the pill

Results of important large studies have received much attention from the press and other mass media. Where the pill is concerned and when the news has been perceived as negative, the effect on users of oral contraceptives has been described as 'pill scares', making women abandon the pill either temporarily or for good. These scares have led to lower use rates, as was the case in the late seventies after publication of the RGCP study which showed an apparent excess mortality from cardio-vascular disease in pill-users over 35 who smoked. As Ketting pointed out, it was not especially the at risk group — the over 35-year-old smokers — who went off the pill, but all age groups together[21].

In 1983, a similar wave of publications appeared in the daily and weekly press following the papers of Pike and colleagues and Vessey and colleagues on the apparent increased risk of breast cancer in certain defined groups of pill-users and an increased relative risk for cancer of the uterine cervix. This second 'pill scare' seems to have had a much smaller effect on pill use than was the case in 1978. As Smith remarked, the newspapers and the doctors panicked, but the women much less[22].

The media, feeling responsible for informing the public, are confronted by the same problem that faces the doctor who counsels: the difficulty of explaining and understanding any epidemiology without dangerous generalisation and half-truths, but with a desired level of vulgarisation so as to be comprehensible.

Several other problems are added to this: in the first place, the preference for negative news, which is believed to possess more novelty value than good news. Thus the 'prevented' deaths due to a lowered incidence of ovarian and endometrial cancer, a very important benefit of oral contraception, have received very little public attention. Secondly, and probably more importantly, there has been a marked lack of follow-up and updating in the developments that have been applied by the manufacturers. For this reason too many women still think that oral contraception will give them heart disease. Most newspapers seriously try to explain the relevant scientific publications to their readers. Other types of publications, women's magazines, for instance, are more inclined to start from individual experiences of users who have had adverse side-effects and then widen the scope of their articles by quoting one or more of the bigger studies on the health effects of oral contraceptives. Understandably, this approach is much more appealing to their readers, but also misleading, because the same readers will not always be able to distinguish the two elements and in consequence they retain a muddled and negative image.

Apart from all this, oral contraceptives have been under fire from those who are opposed to the 'unnatural long-term administration of chemicals', making women solely responsible for contraception and dependent on the medical profession. In such terms, the Feminist Health Movement has expressed its opposition to the pill[23]. In this context, the pill has become a 'peg' on which is put a whole complex of uneasy feelings about all kinds of things in modern society, and an objective approach is hardly to be expected.

Generally speaking, therefore, it is obvious that there is not enough accuracy and unbiased selectivity in media coverage when it comes to the subject of oral contraceptives[24, 25].

Package inserts

Information on oral contraceptives also reaches the users by way of the Patient Package Insert.

This documentation provided by the manufacturers is read with interest by the majority of users[26, 27], but, unfortunately, the nature of the information contained and the format do not necessarily enhance understanding[28, 29]. It has been pointed out[21] that this type of communication does not take into account the educational achievements, high or low, of its receivers. In small print, lists of possible side-effects are given, including warnings about contra-indications. To meet current regulations the inserted information has to be complete and accurate, as the manufacturer is also obliged at the same time to protect himself against legal liability. The result is a selective emphasis on the risks of oral contraceptives — a negative approach presented in a technical way that renders users even more dependent on medical expertise for interpretation.

Again, women cannot be expected to make a balanced judgement with this type of information alone and it has been shown that more extensive and balanced information in the form of leaflets handed out is preferred to package inserts by many users[27].

The informal circuit

The pill, as already observed, is the most widely known and used contraceptive and has also enjoyed an unprecedented attention from the media. As contraception is associated with sexuality and procreation, it can be safely assumed that oral contraceptives figure in countless conversations between relatives, friends, colleagues and neighbours.

Some of the magnitude of this informal communication was traced in the surveys on contraceptives in the five countries in Western Europe, where it was found that about half of the important information was derived from non-professional sources, with family — for instance, discussions between mother and daughter — and friends rating around 20%[2-6].

Undoubtedly, the practical advantages of oral contraceptives play an important part in this type of ubiquitous communication.

As health is the prime concern for choosing or abandoning methods of contraception, negative side-effects of the pill inevitably figure in day-to-day conversations. When directly asked, probably a minority of women actually know someone who has or has had any real disease caused by taking the pill. Where rumour is concerned, even distant cousins or friends or friends one has never met will do because, even in imagination, they are identifiable, non-anonymous people. No doubt countless users, or potential users of the pill are appeased by their doctors, when they are frightened enough by rumours to go for advice.

Nevertheless, this circuit of communication seems to lead its own life and is not compatible with the other available forms of communication on oral contraceptives. Individual experiences of real people are hard to assimilate to relative risks and statistics. Informal communication probably gives a lot of credit to the advantages of the pill, while the disadvantages claimed are inevitably not in correspondence with actual evidence. Thus it is that a 'public view of the pill' is formed. Historically, it is the *vox populi* that has created the perspectives and the image for the pill in the last three decades, and not always scientific advance.

REFERENCES

1. Kay, C. (1980). The happiness pill? *J. Royal Coll. Gen. Pract.*, **30**, 8–19
2. Riphagen, F. E., van der Vurst, J. and Lehert, P. (1984). *Contraception in Italy*. International Health Foundation, Geneva
3. Riphagen, F. E., van der Vurst, J. and Lehert, P. (1985). *Contraception in France*. International Health Foundation, Geneva
4. Riphagen F. E., van der Vurst, J. and Lehert, P. (1985). *Contraception in Great Britain*. International Health Foundation, Geneva
5. Riphagen, F. E., van der Vurst, J. and Lehert, P. (1986). *Contraception in Spain*. International Health Foundation, Geneva
6. Riphagen, F. E., van der Vurst, J. and Lehert, P. (1986). *Contraception in the Federal Republic of Germany*. International Health Foundation, Geneva . (In press)

7. Potts, D. M. and Riphagen, F. E. (1986). *A World Opinion Poll on Oral Contraception.* (In press)
8. The American College of Obstetricians and Gynecologists (1985). *Summary of the Gallup on American Attitudes and Knowledge of Contraception.* Washington
9. Vessey, M. P., Smith, M. A. and Yeates, D. (1986). Return of fertility after discontinuation of oral contraceptives: influence of age and parity. *Br. J. Fam. Plan.*, **ii**, 4
10. Forman, D., Vincent, T. J. and Doll, R. (1986). Cancer of the liver and the use of oral contraceptives. *Br. Med. J.*, **292**, 1357-61
11. Pike, M. C., Henderson, B. E., Krailo, M. D., Duke, A. and Roy, S. (1983). Breast cancer in young women and use of oral contraceptives: possible modifying effect of formulation and age at use. *Lancet*, **2**, 926–30
12. The Centers for Disease Control (1983). Long-term oral contraceptive use and the risk of breast cancer. *J. Am. Med. Assoc.*, **249**, 1591–5
13. Editorial (1985). Another look at the pill and breast cancer. *Lancet*, **ii**, 985–7
14. Vessey, M. P., Lawless, M., McPherson, K. and Yeates, D. (1983). Neoplasia of the cervix uteri and contraception: a possible adverse effect of the pill. *Lancet*, **2**, 930–4
15. Inman, W. H., Vessey, M. P., Westerholm, B. and Engelund, A. (1970). Thromboembolic disease and the steroidal content of oral contraceptives. A report to the Committee on Safety of Drugs. *Br. Med. J.*, **ii**, 203–9
16. RCGP (1977). Royal College of General Practitioners' oral contraception study: Mortality among oral contraceptive users. *Lancet*, **ii**, 727–31
17. Kay, C. R. (1984). Royal College of General Practitioners' oral contraception study: Some recent observations. *Clin. Obstet. Gynaecol.*, **ii**, No. 3, December
18. Vessey, M. P. and Lawless, M. (1984). The Oxford Family Planning Association contraceptive study. *Clin. Obstet. Gynaecol.*, **11**, No. 3, December
19. The Centers for Disease Control (1983). Oral contraceptive use

and the risk of ovarian cancer. *J. Am. Med. Assoc.*, **245**, 1596–9

20. The Centers for Disease Control (1983). Oral contraceptive use and the risk of endometrial cancer. *J. Am. Med. Assoc.*, **249**, 1600–4

21. Ketting, E. (1985). The consumer's interpretation of the risks and benefits of oral contraception. In *Acceptability and Acceptance of Oral Contraception*. International Health Foundation, Geneva

22. Smith, M. (1986). Personal communication

23. Seaman, B. (1980). *The Doctor's Case Against the Pill*. Doubleday, New York

24. Somers, R. L. and Gammeltoft, M. (1976). The impact of liberalized abortion on contraceptive practice in Denmark. *Stud. Fam. Plan.*, **7**, 218–23

25. Smith, M. (1984). Benefits and risks of hormonal contraception-interpretation. In Rolland, R. (ed.) *Advances in Fertility Control and the Treatment of Sterility*, pp 51–6. MTP Press Ltd, Lancaster, Boston and The Hague

26. Fleckenstein, L., Joubert, P., Lawrence, R., Patsner, B., Mazzullo, J. M. and Lasagna, L. (1976). Oral contraceptive patient information. *J. Am. Med. Assoc.*, **235**, 13

27. Mazis, M., Morris, L. A. and Gordon, E. (1978). Patients' attitudes about two forms of printed oral contraceptive information. *Med. Care*, **XVI**, 12

28. Liguori, S. (1978). A quantitative assessment of the readability of PPIs. *Drug Intel. Clin. Pharm.*, **12**, 712–16

29. Casey, F. G., Fluitt, D. M. and Wiatt, A. L. (1983). The patient's understanding of the oral contraceptive Patient Package Insert. *Milit. Med.*, **148**

Chapter 6

The Pill and Women's Health

'The statement that no effective drug can be absolutely safe is understandable and acceptable — but such agents are usually used for the cure of the sick, while the pill is being administered to normal healthy women.' When Greenblatt highlighted, thus, in 1980 the difference between a therapeutic medication and what was basically a 'social' medication, as is the oral contraceptive, he was summarising the dilemma of two decades of its usage by the otherwise healthy population of the developed world. During that time the attitude of the medical profession had become one of concern about the long-term effects of something that in general the female population had clamoured for. Similarly, over the same period the media had instilled, or at least played upon, guilt feelings of women about 'doing something to their bodies' in order to achieve their new-found freedom from the possibility of pregnancy. It had become a widespread feeling that the pill was not natural and that there was a price to pay for the liberation it gave — and in consequence there had been a series of what are now called 'pill scares', when reports of perhaps exaggerated hazards, in the press and communication media, had panicked women into stopping its use. It was, nevertheless, a mass consumption product. For example, in the UK in the five years between 1968 and 1973 the number of married women who had recently had a baby and were then using the pill had doubled. By 1980 over sixty million women world-wide were using it, and yet how it works and what it does to a woman's physiology is to some extent still unknown to medical scientists, as the ramifications of sexual biochemistry are progressively being unravelled.

The question 'How does the pill work?' could be answered at a number of levels by 1980. It was known that both combined (estrogen and progestogen) and other (phasic dosed — see Chapter 7) forms inhibited ovulation and there was evidence that this was achieved because they depressed the pituitary gland's (the hormone release 'controller' at the base of the brain) output of gonadotropins, i.e., the secretory stimulus hormones of the secondary sexual glands, such as the ovary. There is a feedback action of estrogen and progestogen levels which the brain (hypothalamus) detects and if the level is high (e.g., when the pill is taken) then the release of egg cell follicle stimulating hormone (and luteinising hormone) is reduced. It was also known that the hormones of the pill modified tubal (of the uterus) contractions and therefore would affect the transport of an egg if ovulation did occur. They also affected the endometrium (lining wall of the uterus), making implantation unlikely. In addition, the pill altered the character of cervical mucus, rendering it hostile to sperm, and the progestogens of the pill affected the sperm during their transit through the reproductive tract, inhibiting their fertilisation capacity. The ability of the pill, therefore, to make assurance double sure — with regard to contraceptive effect — accounted for its exceptional effectiveness. Very few pharmaceutical compounds have such a predictable and reliable quality as the oral contraceptives.

'Variations in the absorption of these steroids, the variety of metabolic pathways to which they are exposed, differences in patterns of transport and secretion, the interrelations of the feedback between the ovary, the hypothalamus and pituitary, the reduction but not the elimination of the woman's own secretion levels in the presence of the ones she takes by mouth, the fact that the action of progestogens is modified by preceding exposure to oestrogens and the added complexity that, in appropriate doses, oestrogens and progestogens act synergistically — *all make the pharmacokinetics of contraceptive steroids a subject of great complexity*,' wrote Potts (1983), President of Family Health International and previously Medical Adviser to the International Planned Parenthood Federation. He continued: 'Some important questions remain unanswered, particularly in relation to metabolism.'

This, the question of what else the pill does to a woman — apart from its contraceptive effect — had occupied physiologists, biochemists, clinicians and epidemiologists world-wide for the last thirty years, and will probably continue to do so for many a decade more.

Natural steroid hormones bring about widespread sustained and cyclical changes in adult women, from puberty through pregnancy and lactation to the menopause. Not surprisingly, the giving of artificial and extra hormones for prolonged intervals to regulate fertility also brings about extensive changes in the user's physiology. There is evidence that in the early history of man, during the hunter–gatherer stage of evolution, pregnancy intervals of 3–4 years were achieved and sustained by prolonged periods of lactation, which suppressed menstruation and ovulation. The menstrual periods that modern woman experiences, therefore, repeated several hundred times throughout her reproductive life, are thus genuinely an artefect, just as the pill is, too. Modern life in terms of evolution is distinctly artificial.

Evidence about what happens to pill-users has nevertheless accumulated to a greater extent than it has about any other single pharmaceutical substance in current medical usage, but it has at times raised perhaps more questions than it has answered. For example, with regard to the normal physiological changes in women, the study of pill-users over nearly thirty years has dramatically advanced medical knowledge in many fields, whilst opening doors on areas hitherto never explored.

Although the pill may temporarily suppress pituitary function, even after prolonged use ovulation returns, even if in some women there is a delay in return to regular menstruation. The ovaries themselves may thicken their outer lining, but after pill-taking is stopped their response to hormone stimulus, consisting in the production of normal follicles, remains unchanged. Oral contraceptives do not alter the onset of the time of the menopause. Whilst they alter the uterine lining and tubal motility, these too return to normal after cessation of pill use.

Oral contraceptives, like pregnancy and to a lesser extent the menopause, are nevertheless associated with a wide range of metabolic changes. To date, up to 150 different individual metabolic parameters have been measured and been shown to change when a woman takes the pill, but the clinical significance, if any, of many of the alterations is difficult to interpret. Liver changes are sometimes pronounced, thyroid gland secretion changes occur, and blood fat and glucose tolerance levels are altered (similar to, but to a lesser degree than in pregnancy). With regard to the latter change, women taking oral contraceptives show changes in the levels of serum triglyceride, cholesterol, low-density and very-low-density lipoproteins. In general all these tend to be raised, but then a rise in the levels of tri-glycerides and cholesterol also occurs in pregnancy. All these blood fat level changes return to normal shortly after discontinuing use of the pill. Nevertheless, on the whole oral contraceptives seem to alter the fats and proteins in the blood, making those of a fertile woman rather more like those of a man, or at least a woman in an older age group. This in itself has been a major preoccupation of medical scientists trying to explain or rationalise apparent changes in the epidemiology of various diseases in pill-takers, in contrast to non-pill-takers, over the last twenty years.

The history of oral contraceptives has therefore been the accumulation of important knowledge *following* their widespread use. In the UK and a few other countries there is a system for the voluntary recording by physicians of adverse side-effects of medication, but rarely more than 15% of significant events are reported. In practice, it is also exceptionally difficult to follow up large numbers of contraceptive users and to find out what happens to them over many years. Modern populations are mobile; divorce, remarriage, change of name or life-style, different medication regimes and occupational or social hazards all make the human being a different 'animal' to study from that of the laboratory. Similarly, retrospective studies which seek a disease's pattern of incidence from historical surveys of habits or medication regimes that are remembered are equally fallible in proving, satisfactorily, any demonstrable cause and effect. Taking the pill as an example, there have been at least four major changes in its dosage regime in the last twenty years, so studies that set out to test its long-term effect are inevitably bedevilled by the fact that few women indeed have taken the 'same' pill for any prolonged period of time.

Unfortunately, all reported epidemiological studies of pill-users have become the focus of media attention and 'instant' interpretation, which has often been misinterpretation. Not surprisingly therefore, as has been noted, associations based on the absorption of misinformation have perhaps predominated in the views and attitudes of women in the last two decades, without the benefit of sober interpretation, understanding and wisdom of perspective. Alarm has too often been the sound, when reassurance would have been more appropriate.

Whilst the pill-maker deals in concern, initially about reliability and then subsequently about long-term hazards, the epidemiologist deals in probabilities and administrators have to make 'political' decisions. Drug regulatory authorities have to respond to many different pressures and in the last twenty years have become trapped in having to ask for a proof of safety of a drug before it is marketed, and logically this is impossible. Trials on relatively few otherwise healthy individuals can never predict the likely outcome of widespread use by a population made up of the obese, anorexic, ill, sporting, smoking, alcohol-using, accident-prone and genetically defective members of the so-called 'normal' society. In the last analysis, every new drug is an experiment on our own species. All that can be done is to establish a testing system which takes all reasonable and prudent steps to reduce foreseeable risks: the unknown is, of its nature, unpredictable and there will always be a hazard when new chemical substances are introduced for protracted use, as in contraception.

In 1970 Djerassi estimated that it would take up to ten years and cost ten to twenty million dollars to introduce a new method of contraception, that would, prior to release, satisfy the then required criteria of the US Food and Drug Administration. Today the cost would be as high as fifty million dollars. It is just as well that a decade earlier the first forms of the pill were able to be marketed without the restrictive requirements of today, for the proof of its safety in such idealistic terms is still awaited and it would never have been released. Hazards did emerge in the first twenty years of its use, hazards that were entirely unpredictable in the light of current knowledge at the time of its launch, but then by learning from these the pill's continual evolution has been assured. Oral contraceptives have become a model for the post-marketing surveillance of any drug.

With hindsight the introduction of the pill could have been more rationally engineered, but there was nothing whatsoever in the early use of oral contraceptives that was out of step with the stage of evolution of drug regulatory requirements reached at the time, in either the USA or the UK.

Chapter 7

The Evolution of the Pill and the Surveillance of its Effects

The clinical history of oral contraception — that is its application in the human being as distinct from the pharmaceutical history of development in the laboratory — evolved from the work in the USA in 1940 of Sturgis and Albright, who employed injections of estradiol benzoate (estrogen) every few days through a woman's menstrual cycle in an effort to inhibit ovulation and thus 'cure' dysmenorrhea (painful periods). However, ovulation escaped every other month, making this regime, complicated and uncomfortable enough as it was, ineffective. Robert Greenblatt, Professor of Endocrinology at Georgia University, Atlanta, two years later recommended daily suppositories of stilboestrol as a treatment, with some success, and others — Lyons in 1943, and Hamblen and colleagues in 1947 — used an oral estrogen from day 5 to day 25 of the women patients' cycles with similar success. In 1953–4 Greenblatt again tried out these oral estrogens, in a continuous regime of descending dosage with the interposition of several days of an oral progestogen to induce menstruation, and reported this in the *American Journal of Obstetrics and Gynecology* as successfully suppressing ovulation for over a year. The concept of a cyclical form of medication with varying dosages of hormones was born. Thus it was on this work that Rock, Garcia and Pincus based their trial in Puerto Rico when they used the newly available and potent progestogen, norethisterone (unknowingly 'contaminated' with the estrogen, mestranol). The dosage chosen for the first commercial pill, Enavid, was thus almost a hit and miss decision — there had to be enough progestogen to control the woman's cycle and enough estrogen when the mestranol was added to ensure pregnancy did not occur. In consequence, whilst it is now known that it was an overdose, it was then thought to be reasonably safe. There was, however, in 1959 a daily dose of nearly 10 mg of progestogen and 150 microgram of estrogen being administered in the classic pill — nearly a hundred times more active substance than was necessary, but it took nearly twenty years to find that out.

Two years after Enavid appeared, Ortho Pharmaceuticals obtained a licence for their preparation Ortho-Novum (USA), with the same 10 mg of norethisterone but less than half (60 microgram) the estrogen component, mestranol, and similarly in 1961 Schering brought out their pill with only 50 microgram of the estrogen component. At the same time Greenblatt was working on a further sophistication of the reduced dosage regime in a sequential pattern. 'I questioned the need of a progestogen for 21 days . . . for if oestrogens alone inhibit ovulation, why not use a progestogen only in the latter part of the cycle?' he wrote. 'Using an "in tandem" regimen (oestrogen from day 9–19, progestogen from day 20–24) this proved quite effective and acceptable to patients . . . especially in women in whom the combination pill had decreased their libido.' Thus in 1965 the sequential pill was invented, as the second generation of oral contraceptives.

What was actually happening clinically was that women were experiencing many unwanted side-effects from the high estrogen and the other progestogen hormone dosages they were taking. Some were trivial and others, as time was to prove, were quite dangerous. Nausea, vomiting, breast engorgement, breakthrough bleeding, weight gain, headaches, skin changes, greasy hair, visual disturbances and loss of libido were leading to many women abandoning the pill. There was a constant move, therefore, by pharmaceutical manufacturers to reduce these side-effects, by cutting down the dose and trying new synthetic hormones in order to produce a more acceptable product.

In 1966 the first progestogen-only pill was marketed, for women with unacceptable side-effects from estrogen, but it inevitably caused breakthrough bleeding problems and suffered a certain incidence of failure as a contraceptive, i.e., pregnancy.

There were two major set-backs in the evolution of the pill, the tailoring of its dose, and the development of new steroids, that occurred firstly in the United Kingdom and secondly in the USA. In 1961 Dr. W. M. Jordan, a GP in Suffolk (UK), wrote to the *Lancet* reporting that in one of the patients for whom he had been prescribing Enavid as a treatment for endometriosis (a menstrual tissue aberration with spread to the pelvic organs) a pulmonary embolus (clot in the blood vessels of the lung) had occurred. The Royal College of General Practitioners set up a monitoring survey of pill-takers (that has continued its work since 1964 to date) and by 1969, through this and the Oxford Study of Family Planning Association patients conducted by Vessey, Inman and Doll, sufficient suspicion had been aroused to associate venous thrombosis and myocardial infarction (coronary thrombosis) with the high dosage of hormonal steroids being taken in the pill. As a result the UK Committee on Safety of Medicines recommended that the pill should have a maximum level of 50 microgram of estrogen. The pill and thrombosis had become incontrovertibly linked in the minds of scientists, clinicians and public alike.

In 1972, Schering introduced a thirty microgram estrogen pill (Eugynon 30) and two years later Parke-Davis brought out their twenty microgram preparation (Loestrin), in the light of the RCGP findings and those of another survey being conducted at Walnut Creek in the USA. Altogether, by the early 1970s there were 46 000 women being studied by 1400 GPs in the Royal College survey, and the Oxford FPA and Walnut Creek surveys studied another 17 000 women each.

By 1976, therefore, from these surveys there was a general consensus that the estrogenic effects of the pill were firmly linked with thrombo-embolic events, but the association of compounding risk factors such as age, obesity, family history, and cigarette smoking was yet to emerge. A year later the RCGP study suggested that there was a further correlation between hypertension (high blood-pressure) in women taking the pill and its progestogen content. Because of these links intense study of what effect, if any, oral contraceptives have on blood-fat (lipid) metabolism then became vital research. Since it was held that low blood concentration of high density lipoprotein (HDL) cholesterol and the occurrence of coronary heart disease were associated, the effects of the various steroid hormones on HDL were rapidly assessed. Bradley in 1978 concluded that progestogen tends to lower HDL and estrogen to raise it, thus the particular effect of a given oral contraceptive on blood fats depends on that pill's progestogen: estrogen ratio.

Meanwhile, however, the steroids being used, the dosages and the ratios of one hormone to another were being constantly changed, and reduced progressively. Phased types of preparations, sequential dosages and new steroids were being investigated, and the 'pill' which the average woman was taking in the 1970s was a very different one from the earlier 'classics'. Indeed, by 1979 the daily steroid dose had dropped from 10 mg of progestogen (as norethisterone) to 0.15 mg (as levonorgestrel), and the estrogen from 150 microgram (as mestranol) to 30 microgram (as ethinyl estradiol). Retrospective surveys of the pill and assumed effects over long-term use were therefore being rendered almost meaningless, since women were no longer taking the same pill; it was history, not prediction, that was emerging.

Thus, when several eminent commentators on statistics related to contraception (Tietze in 1980 and Wiseman in 1981) pointed out the discrepancy between an increase in the use of the pill over the previous decade and a *decrease* in mortality rates for cardio-vascular disease in women, it threw the correlations that had previously been made into dispute. Nevertheless, the research into the metabolic effects of the hormones, the epidemiological studies, the induced caution in clinicians in prescribing the pill to 'assumed-risk' women, and the changes in the steroids themselves, as well as the dosage, actually and inevitably led to an improvement in the health and the surveillance of it, in women who used the pill. The 'thrombosis-story' may have been a set-back — as the first widely reported scare it had led to an accelerated downward trend in the use of the pill, for as one authority put it 'the women's press were more influential than the Pope in decreasing oral contraceptive use' — but it was a gain in medical knowledge.

The second major set-back that occurred in the same decade proved to be equally disputatious, but less of a gain to medical science.

Soon after their introduction in the 1960s Enavid and Ortho-Novum were followed by other contraceptive steroids. Many of these were closely related to norethisterone, and others, such as medroxy progesterone acetate, megestrol acetate and chlormadinone acetate, were analogues, or 'look-alikes', of the 17-acetoxyprogesterone type. A third and more potent type of compound belonged to the family of '18-homo-steroids' and one of these, levonorgestrel, discovered by Schering, proved to be the most potent (and therefore usable in smaller dosage) and successful progestogen synthesised up to date. In the mid-sixties the licensing authorities were faced with concern about the testing of these new products (bearing in mind the cardio-vascular disease controversy over the products already released) and it was decided by the American Food and Drug Administration that as well as monkey and other animal tests, tests should also be carried out on the beagle dog as a 'non-rodent toxicological model of preference'. Diczfalusy, writing later about this decision, which was also taken up by virtually all the other national drug regulatory agencies, said: 'The almost incredible part of the story is that extensive large-scale beagle studies were requested to be conducted with a variety of progestogens in the virtual absence of any information about the pharmacokinetic and pharmacodynamic behaviour of these progestogens in the canine species.' A disaster of monumental proportions thus occurred, for when prolonged administration of certain progestogens was carried out on beagle dogs it resulted in the development of mammary (breast) nodules, and sometimes even of tumours of frightening appearance. The FDA thus advised that such steroids should be removed from the market and the public heard the story of 'breast cancer and the pill' — never to forget it, though unaware of the true scientific significance of the findings.

In consequence, the second major scare story emerged, to be re-echoed in 1981 when Pike claimed from a survey of women pill-users in California to have detected a higher than normal incidence of breast tumours (information which later was disputed) and several useful steroid compounds (e.g., chlormadinone acetate and megestrol acetate, the former of which is still being tested by the World Health Organisation) were shelved. The dust was slow to settle, although it is established now that progesterone causes mammary tumours in dogs most probably because in the canine species (in contradistinction to others) progestational agents induce a marked excess of the secretion of growth hormone, something which does not occur in humans. The beagle dog, therefore, is an entirely unsuitable animal for the assessment of carcinogenicity of progestational agents, and since this discovery the American, British, Swedish and other drug regulatory agencies have withdrawn their requirement of tests to be performed on this animal. Diczfalusy in 1979 summarised the effects of this historic set-back as: 'The damage to the field of steroidal contraception has been a significant one, leading to a major discouragement of the pharmaceutical industry and to a drastic reduction in the volume of their research on new contraceptive agents.'

Nevertheless, following on the World Health Organisation recommendation of 1978 that 'it is advisable to use the lowest possible effective and acceptable dose of steroid contraceptive preparations so as to minimise any potential risk', the pharmaceutical manufacturers continued to develop the preparations they already had. By phasing the dosage to reduce the total hormone taken in any one cycle, Schering, for example, with their tri-phasic preparation (also introduced subsequently by Wyeth), which had been developed over a period since 1974, released in 1980 a pill preparation that had in it less than 1% of the daily dose of the active hormones that had been administered twenty years earlier. The pill had evolved, not in a story that was trouble-free, but in a way that nevertheless brought progressively greater than ever 'safety', as well as unimpaired security, to contemporary women.

Chapter 8

The Mechanism of the Pill

J. Guillebaud

Oral contraception evolved as both the natural physiological 'mechanisms' of fertility within the body became better understood and the synthetic manufacturing of drugs to 'interfere' with these mechanisms became available. Both of these areas have therefore been under constant review for well over the last half-century and will probably remain so for the foreseeable future, since the science of contraception is only part of the quest for further knowledge about the function of the human body.

The current status of knowledge in the regulation of fertility is enormously advanced, by comparison with even less than a decade ago — not least, though perhaps ironically — by the advances brought about by the ever-increasing success of treatment regimes for *infertility*; the 'test-tube' or *in-vitro* fertilisation regime, for example. Nevertheless, there are still areas that await a breakthrough, and today's knowledge of human physiology will certainly be outdated as time goes by. What is known today soon becomes history in such a rapidly advancing science.

In the light of present knowledge, however, the processes of menstruation, ovulation, conception and implantation are all better understood than ever before and a summary of what is known points to possible future developments in the science of control, i.e., contraception.

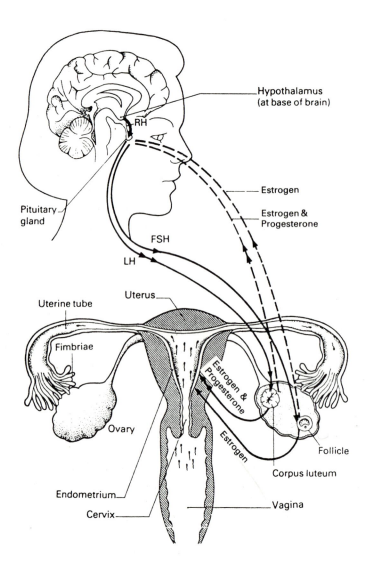

Figure 1 The female reproductive system: control of the menstrual cycle. Single arrowhead relates to events in the first half of the cycle (follicular phase). Double arrowheads relate to the second half (luteal phase). Dotted lines show feedback effects. (From: Guillebaud, J. (1984). *The Pill*. Oxford University Press, Oxford)

THE FOLLICULAR PHASE

In order to start each new cycle, a special hormone called the releasing hormone (RH) is produced in the base of the brain in discrete bursts or pulses about every ninety minutes. It travels to the pituitary gland and causes it to release follicle-stimulating hormone (FSH). FSH travels in the blood to the ovaries. Its main action, as its name implies, is to stimulate the growth of some of the many thousands of follicles which are contained in each ovary. Follicles are tiny, thick-walled, fluid-filled egg-sacs, each lined by a layer of cells which are capable of producing hormones, and also containing an immature egg cell (oocyte). FSH usually stimulates about twenty of these follicles to grow, and also causes the lining cells to start to manufacture estrogen and release it into the blood. One particular follicle in one or other ovary is stimuted to grow and to 'ripen' more than all the others. Its egg cell is also maturing, ready to be released and, should it get the chance, to be fertilised.

Estrogens are the fundamentally female hormones which influence the whole body, producing rounded contours, breast development, and many other features of femininity. They also stimulate the uterus to grow its new lining to replace the one that was shed at the previous menstrual period. The lining is made of many glands, set in several layers of cells which also contain arteries and veins. Estrogen makes the glands grow and the layers of intervening cells increase.

Meanwhile the rising levels of estrogen in the blood have been having a most important effect back on the base of the brain and the pituitary gland. This is known as 'negative feedback'.

In general terms, negative feedback means that if the level of a hormone in the blood goes up, the level of the stimulating hormone which *caused* it to go up is made to go *down*.

In the menstrual cycle, this means for example:

up ↑ estrogen in blood causes *down* ↓ FSH.

The opposite is also true:

down ↓ estrogen in blood causes *up* ↑ FSH.

By about the thirteenth day of a standard 28-day cycle the stimulated follicles have produced a rise of estrogen in the blood to a peak
level up to six times higher than it was on the first day. By negative
feedback this has caused the level of the stimulating hormone FSH to
drop. Now a most interesting and crucially different thing happens.
Once the amount of estrogen reaching the pituitary gland gets to
a critical level, it releases into the bloodstream a sudden surge of
luteinising hormone (LH). Thus, the *rise* in estrogen is now causing a
rise of a hormone from the pituitary. This is called 'positive feedback'.

This large amount of LH is conveyed by the blood to the active
ovary, the one containing the largest follicle, now a 'blister' bulging
the surface of the ovary and about two centimetres in diameter. The
main job of this surge of LH is to cause the follicle to burst, resulting
in ovulation and the release of a now mature and fertilisable egg. If all
goes well, this is picked up by the fimbriae of the uterine tube and
transported towards the uterus. (As this occurs some women notice in

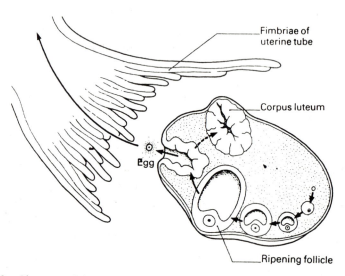

Figure 2 Close-up of the ovary to show the growth of follicles and formation of
the corpus luteum after egg-release. (From: Guillebaud, J. (1984). *The Pill*. Oxford
University Press, Oxford)

their lower abdomen, on one or other side, a variable amount of pain which is given the German name 'Mittelschmerz'.)

Once the egg has been released, the follicle collapses and becomes that bright yellow body, the corpus luteum. Along with the change in colour of the cells lining its wall there is a change in what they do. As well as continuing to produce estrogen, for the first time these luteal cells start to manufacture and release into the blood a new hormone called progesterone.

THE LUTEAL PHASE

Progesterone, like estrogen, has effects all over the body and, for instance, is responsible for the slight rise in body temperature during the second half of the cycle which is the basis for the temperature method of family planning. But its main effect is on the lining of the uterus, to prepare it for a pregnancy. Indeed the word 'progesterone' means 'pro-gestation: in favour of childbearing'. It thickens the lining of the uterus still further and causes its glands to release a nutritious fluid. After implantation, which if a sperm successfully fertilises an egg is about five days after its release, the embryo produces human chorionic gonadotropin (hCG). This hormone exactly copies the action of LH from the pituitary and so prolongs the life of the corpus luteum, ensuring that it continues to produce sufficient progesterone and estrogen. As long as these hormones continue to be produced by the ovary, there will be no menstrual flow and the embryo can remain secure within the lining of the uterus. A second effect of these two hormones, working in concert, is to lower the amounts of LH and FSH released from the pituitary by the more usual negative feedback process. This is important, as it prevents any more surges of LH.

If, however, a sperm fails to reach the egg on its way down the tube, the egg dies at a maximum of forty-eight hours after ovulation. For reasons which are still not clear, the corpus luteum abruptly ceases to function twelve to fourteen days after it was first formed, unless hCG from a developing embryo dictates differently. There is therefore a rapid fall in the levels of both estrogen and progesterone. This has two results: first, by negative feedback, the amount of RH coming from the base of the brain to the pituitary increases and therefore the amount of FSH released increases. When this extra FSH in the blood reaches the ovaries, another group of twenty or so follicles is stimulated to grow, one of them being destined to release its egg during the *next* normal menstrual cycle. Second, the sudden fall in the levels of both estrogen and progesterone in the bloodstream reaching the uterus causes local changes in its now thick lining which lead to it being shed during a normal menstrual period. How heavy and how long the bleeding during the first few days of the next cycle is varies considerably. Prostaglandins are involved in this process: one of their effects is to ensure that the uterus contracts to expel the blood, but this can also cause menstrual cramping pain (dysmenorrhea), which can be severe in some women.

'Estrogen' is in fact a family of hormones, the most important member of which in the menstrual cycle is estradiol. The surge of LH is accompanied by a smaller surge of FSH. Another hormone from the pituitary gland, called prolactin, is involved; and the whole cycle can be affected by quite different hormones, such as those from the thyroid gland, as well as by the nervous system.

THE MECHANISM OF ORAL CONTRACEPTION

In summary, therefore, with oral contraception it can be seen that so long as there are reasonably high levels of the two hormones, estrogen and progesterone, the pulses of releasing hormone from the base of the brain are suppressed and the pituitary gland is kept inactive (by negative feedback). This prevents:

(a) release of sufficient FSH to ripen any follicles in preparation for egg-release;

(b) any surges of LH, without which the actual process of release of an egg is impossible.

These results are also regularly produced by the high levels of both the natural hormones during the second half of the normal menstrual cycle and throughout any pregnancy.

The principle ways by which the usual combined pill operates to prevent pregnancy are shown in Figure 3 and Table 1. The main effect is to stop the normal hormone changes of the menstrual cycle and hence prevent both maturing of follicles and ovulation — items 1 and 2 in Table 1. However, there are several back-up mechanisms to make pregnancy unlikely even if egg-release does occur. The mucus which normally flows from the cervix in the middle of the cycle and at that time is easily penetrated by sperm is transformed by the hormone progestogen into a scanty, thick material which produces a quite different barrier to sperm. There are also changes in the lining of the uterus which seem to make it less able to support and nourish a fertilised egg. Finally, it is thought that the tubes may perhaps function less well in conveying the egg towards the uterus, perhaps making it less likely to survive even if it were fertilised.

Table 1 How the combined pills prevent pregnancy. (The more +s means the greater the effect)

	'Ordinary' combined pills
1 Reduced FSH therefore follicles stopped from ripening and egg from maturing	++++
2 LH surge stopped so no egg-release	++++
3 Cervical mucus changed into a barrier to sperm	+++
4 Lining of uterus made less suitable for implantation of an embryo	+++
5 Uterine tubes perhaps affected so that they do not transport egg so well (uncertainty about this)	+
Expected pregnancy rate per 100 women using the pill method for one year (compare use of *no method* = 80–90)	0.1–1

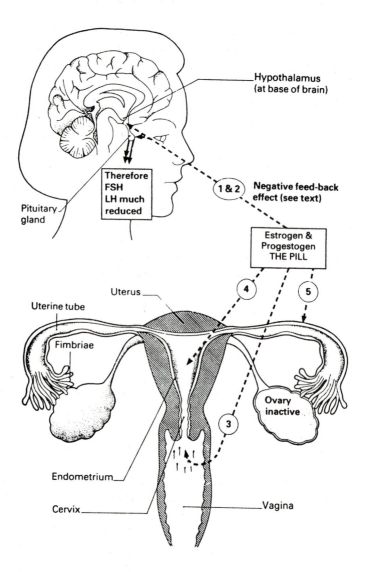

Figure 3 How the combined pill prevents pregnancy. Numbers 1–5 are the contraceptive effects of the combined pill as shown in Table 1. (From: Guillebaud, J. (1984). *The Pill*. Oxford University Press, Oxford)

EFFECTIVENESS AGAINST PREGNANCY

There is no more effective reversible method of fertility control than the combined pill. This is probably because its back-up systems can operate even if the prime effect of preventing release of an egg from the ovary should fail. But failures do occur, for two reasons: failures of the method (which are rare) and failures of the user (forgetting tablets — not so rare). If these two causes of failure are added together, the total failure rate can be as high as two per 100 women-years (i.e., if a hundred women used the pill for a year, two of them should expect to get pregnant). For healthy women who take their pills absolutely regularly at the same time every day, the failure rate is reduced about tenfold, to as low as 0.1 per 100 women-years. This means less than one pregnancy among 1000 users per year.

When the pill is taken the normal menstrual cycle is abolished. Just so long as sufficient of the artificial estrogen and progestogen of the pill are in the bloodstream there will be no bleeding from the uterus. However, most women like to see some kind of period, as regular reassurance that the pill is working. It is also held to be better to reduce the monthly intake of artificial hormones to a minimum, and to give the pituitary and ovaries a break from time to time from the suppressing action of the synthetic hormones. For these reasons, and *only for these reasons*, most systems of pill-taking include a six- or seven-day break every twenty-eight days. The effect of thus cutting off the supply of pill hormones is to *imitate* the fall in the levels in the bloodstream of their natural equivalents at the end of a normal cycle. This causes shedding of the rather thinner lining of the uterus which the pill's hormones have produced during the previous twenty-one days. Because the lining is different, its shedding usually leads to less bleeding, often darker in colour, than in a normal menstrual period. It is also a lot less likely to be painful. As these are in reality *substitute periods*, they are often more accurately called *hormone withdrawal bleeds*.

Thus the use of the oral contraceptive formulations currently available suppresses natural menstruation, imitates the role of the corpus luteum, influences the pituitary by feedback mechanisms, alters the function of cervical mucus and prevents the maturation of ovarian follicles. Fertility control is by no means a simple matter, and it is therefore not surprising that the search continues for either better alternatives or even more precisely targeted preparations.

Bibliography

Guillebaud, J. (1984). *The Pill*. Oxford University Press, Oxford

Chapter 9

The Pill in Perspective

'. . . as in the case of every other problem regarding human life, one must look beyond partial perspectives — whether biological or psychological, demographic or sociological . . .'
Pope Paul VI, *Humanae Vitae*, 25 July, 1968

Hormonal contraceptives are the only genuine 20th century addition to family planning. Condoms, spermicides, vaginal diaphragms, intrauterine devices and male and female sterilisation were all known and used by the end of the 19th century. More significantly, the pill is the only method of contraception to be derived from a scientific understanding of reproductive biology and, not surprisingly, it is the method of contraception which has caused the most profound re-appraisal of the stresses and strains of reproduction on an individual woman and provided the greatest challenge to existing social norms.

Of all the products of modern technology the pill is the most paradoxical. The pill as a possibility of oral contraception using ovarian hormones was accurately described in the 1920s and, had it been developed a few years earlier, it would have become an over-the-counter medication. Once established, like aspirin, it would have remained off prescription and probably acquired a better image. As it is, oral contraceptive pills were first used clinically exactly thirty years ago and since that time they have been taken by something over 100 million people, about 60 million users at the present time. Use grew in the 1960s and 1970s, when epidemiologists and clinicians knew least about its long-term side-effects, yet popularity has declined in the 1980s just as the pill has been demonstrated to have some protective effect against two common reproductive cancers. How should the user view the pill after thirty years of human experience? Socially, oral contraceptives have been perceived as the trigger to the sexual revolution, but was it the cause or merely a symbol?

Over the past thirty years key social issues and problems of health and population growth have worsened. Thirty years ago there were 2500 million people in the world. Today, there are over 5000 million. By happenstance the excess of births over deaths is approximately in step with the calendar year — 86 million more births than deaths in 1986, 87 million extra in 1987 and so forth. India alone adds a million a month to its already out of control population. With half the world's population below the age of marriage and more and more women at risk for pregnancy every year, it is possible more mothers will die in childbirth in the remaining years of the 20th century than at any comparable interval during history.

In the USA the social problems of uncontrolled fertility are no less formidable. One American teenager falls pregnant every thirty seconds and, overall, 40% of American girls will have at least one pregnancy before they turn twenty. The nation spends $16 000 million a year supporting children conceived by teenagers although six out of seven were not intended and almost half of all teenage pregnancies end in abortion.

The past twenty-five years have been a unique experience in the history of technology where scientific advances have been associated with reduction in the number of contraceptive choices available to solve key problems of health and population growth. The United States has less spermicides and fewer IUDs available than twenty-five years ago. Although some IUDs remain approved by the US Food and Drug Administration (FDA), IUDs are no longer for sale in the USA, as a consequence of problems surrounding product liability. America is facing a contraceptive Dunkirk and an American couple can get a wider choice of contraceptives in a so-called developing country such as Mexico, than in Texas or California. Throughout the world, new methods of contraception are coming along slowly and no method is likely to replace oral contraceptives in the foreseeable future.

Haberlandt had foreseen the possibility of oral contraception in the 1920s, Makepeace, Dempsey and Astwood demonstrated that progesterone inhibited ovulation in the late 1930s and the human use of progesterone began in the late 1940s. In 1951 M. C. Chang began experiments in rabbits, using the new synthetic hormones C. Djerassi (norethindrone) and F. D. Colton (norethynodrel) had synthesised. The first human results were reported by Rock, Pincus and Garcia in 1956, when it was shown that an oral contraceptive could be devised that imitated the natural suppression of ovulation found during pregnancy and lactation. No drug was as wanted, proved so effective, offered such a biologically appropriate solution, became so well studied and yet has remained so misunderstood as the oral contraceptive.

The use of progestogens by themselves is associated with breakthrough bleeding and the early investigators soon added small doses of estrogen, producing the classic combined pill. While necessary and convenient, it was a change that narrowed the perspective of all concerned from the slow, important cycles of pregnancy and lactational amenorrhea to the more immediate short-term events of the menstrual cycle. But it we are to think about the pill's real impact then we must return to the life-long perspective on fertility and pause to ask what type of animal homo sapiens really is.

We are a unique primate for whom biological evolution has concealed the time of ovulation and maximum fertility in the female and who practises a universal social tabu of covering up the genitals in public. From a biological point of view these are relatively recent attributes, which help distinguish us from all other apes and are something to do with the type of long-term sexual paired bonding essential to an animal that develops a helpless infant that remains totally dependent on its parents for at least one-tenth of its life and takes one-quarter to one-third of its life span to learn to live as an independent adult capable of reproducing itself. Whether the dissociation of sex from ovulation is an adaptation to our particular pattern of family life, as Symonds suggests, or its origin, as Morris argues, may never be decided as the key changes occurred hundreds of thousands of years ago and fossils do not show emotion. Whatever the details of the evolutionary process, over 90% of human life on earth was spent in hunter-food gathering societies whose physiology and social structure were profoundly different from those of the agricultural, urban and industrialised communities that have made up the last ten thousand years of history and prehistory. As we have seen, women in hunter-gathering societies spent most of their lives pregnant or lactating and menstruation was a rare event. The pill certainly gave us back long intervals of suppressed ovulation.

The pill dissociated contraception from coitus, making it an acceptable and easy-to-use contraceptive. Neither did we have to expose our genitals literally or metaphorically to use the method: no one ever discussed their prowess at coitus interruptus at a cocktail party but women and men, from the late 1960s onwards, have been able to discuss oral contraceptives. The very name, 'the pill', was evocative of the change it has wrought.

Lacking a biological perspective society compared the situation with the previous decade or with the previous century, but not with the environment in which homo sapiens had evolved. The world was not yet ready to understand how truly natural was the pill; instead, many sincere people saw it as an invitation to promiscuity and a threat to family living.

Historically, the pill promised to make a fractured world whole, but to those whose standards were to merely re-emphasise the day before yesterday's norms it did indeed appear revolutionary. Even today it is difficult to recall that when Pincus, Rock and Garcia first published on the pill any form of contraception was *illegal* in Massachusetts. To understand what the pill offered to human society and family life we need to go back, not a century, but ten thousand years.

Despite the current population explosion we are almost the slowest breeding animal in the zoo. We mature even more gradually than our primate cousins and, like them, we are a non-seasonally breeding animal in which pregnancies are spaced by long intervals of anovulation associated with breastfeeding. Chimpanzees, which have an identical physiology, have their pregnancies between four and six years apart, the orang-utan up to eight years. The Bush people of the Kalahari desert, who are hunters and food-gatherers, have four to five live-born children in a lifetime, on average forty-four months apart. They have never seen a contraceptive but breastfeed their babies up to four times an hour and their natural rate of population growth is to double their numbers every three hundred years. Over a lifetime, in such a community, the overwhelming majority of sexual acts take place when the woman is *not* ovulating. By comparison, the average woman in Pakistan has a total fertility rate of 6.2 and the population of the country doubles in twenty-eight years. In Kenya women can expect to have an average of eight children in a lifetime and the country doubles its population in a mere eighteen years. It is not just that modern medicine has reduced infant mortality but changing patterns of breastfeeding mean many more acts of coitus are likely to occur at or near ovulation. The pill, by suppressing ovulation for years on end, takes us back to the 'world' we evolved to enjoy and exploit. Civilised living, by lowering the age of puberty, altering patterns of breastfeeding and reducing infant mortality, has made contraception a necessity.

It has been suggested that oral contraceptives were 'approved for marketing without adequate testing or study'[1]. In reality, oral contraceptives were tested as well, or as poorly, as any other drug marketed at that time. It was the 19th century Comstock laws forbidding contraceptive sales in Massachusetts that forced early trials on oral contraceptives to be undertaken in Puerto Rico. The pioneers of contraception did set up an excellent perspective study of 10 000 users and 10 000 controls, but lack of funding and lack of insight by those less close to the pill slowly eroded this promising beginning.

In 1963 the FDA assembled a group of consultants to review reports of thrombosis among pill-users, but the then available data were ambiguous. In 1966 the FDA Advisory Committee under Prof. Louis Hellman recommended a study 'of as many as 30 000 women for as long as ten years'. In fact, the most important studies were eventually carried out in Britain, where general practice, nationwide vital statistics and fewer pressures by the funding agency to revise studies as they went along created a better climate for long-term research.

Three large perspective cohort studies, and many case-control studies, have now documented the long-term risks and benefits of oral contraceptives more fully than for practically any other drug. During the 1960s and early 1970s it was demonstrated that the pill had a number of rare but serious adverse effects, including the possibility of death due to myocardial infarction, stroke or thrombo-embolic disease. Beneficial effects, of their nature, took longer and were more difficult to demonstrate: it is easier both to understand and document a death due, say, to myocardial infarctional disease than it is to trace and validate a death that did *not* take place because, for example, a woman did *not* develop ovarian cancer. It also happened that most adverse effects occurred during contraceptive use and few, if any, persisted for long intervals after discontinuing the pill, while beneficial effects often took some years to manifest themselves, although they have now been shown to persist for ten or fifteen years — and possibly for a lifetime — after stopping oral contraceptives.

More particularly, death or sickness due to a side-effect hits the headlines and — in the Western world — the law courts, while beneficial effects cannot be individualised. The package insert required by the US FDA in every cycle of oral contraceptives provides a dismal catalogue of possible and proven side-effects but specifically excludes any reference to beneficial effects. In the 1970s US Congressman Nelson had well publicised hearings on the adverse effects of the pill, but no one has thought of moving similarly public hearings on the beneficial effects in the 1980s.

Certainly, all forms of hormonal contraception have had a stormy, emotional history and sincere efforts to put its many benefits and risks into perspective have not always been very successful. Animal as well as human findings about contraception are consistently mis-interpreted. To take a single example, the injectable contraceptive, Depo-Provera, is not available in the United States because, in very high doses, it has given rise to tumours in a handful of beagle dogs and rhesus monkeys, although there is no evidence from more than a million users that the same risk applies to human beings. By contrast, the use of periodic abstinence (the Billings method of natural family planning or mucous method), which requires no drugs or devices, has had a very smooth ride in the press and amongst the medical profession. However, there is much stronger and more consistent evidence that the systematic and artificial separation of the time of intercourse from the time of ovulation increases the risk of abnormal offspring in experimental animals than there is that contraceptive hormones give cancer in experimental animals. The biological vision in hormonal contraceptives is often blurred.

The epidemiological perspective is just as confused. Epidemiology is a difficult science: confounding variables are common even in the best designed study, and on the whole epidemiologists are cautious people. For a relationship to be accepted as causal it is generally useful to have more than one study, preferably in different places, each demonstrating the same trend, and it is especially convincing if there is a dose-response relationship. Of course, any relationship must be both biologically plausible and related in time to the treatment. For example, there is probably a stronger relationship between the number of telegraph poles and the number of heart attacks among men in a community, than there is between the number of women taking pills and the number of heart attacks amongst women — the telegraph poles, however, fail to meet the criteria of causality or biological plausibility.

In the late 1960s Sir Alan Parkes posed the basic issue concerning contraceptive safety, 'It is always difficult to prove a negative and impossible to do so in advance. In fact, we face the dilemma that no woman should be kept on the pill for twenty years, until, in fact, a substantial number have been kept on the pill for twenty years.' We may even have to expand this cautious statement to cover two generations — the user and her offspring. Fortunately, we now have a great deal of data that extends over decades of use: everything from ear wax to gallbladder disease and from rheumatism to liver cancer has been the subject of special studies and work is now focusing on subgroups of users, such as the risk of breast cancer in women who used the pill before age 25. Children born to women exposed to artificial ovarian hormones during pregnancy or lactation are now being followed up through puberty and beyond. The World Health Organisation (WHO) and Family Health International (FHI) are completing a study

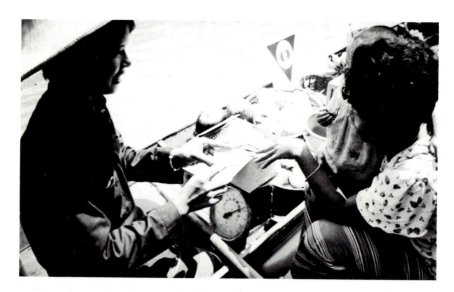

Figure 1 Contraceptives are distributed in many different ways. This woman is selling them from her boat in Bangkok's floating market

in Israel of women exposed to steroids in pregnancy and, in Thailand, of children born to mothers who used Depo-Provera during pregnancy or breastfeeding; no adverse findings have appeared to date.

Most early assessment of pill risks and benefits traded the health benefits of preventing unwanted pregnancies against the direct adverse effects of cardio-vascular disease. However, this type of comparison is inadequate for handling our new understanding of side-effects, which may extend over a significant proportion of a woman's lifetime. FHI has devised an objective way of comparing risks and benefits by developing a computer program to calculate the effect of using the pill for five years, continuously at specified ages, on the overall expectation of life. In building this model every known adverse risk and benefit of the pill was scrutinised although, in the end, only those listed in Table 1 were shown to make a significant effect.

It is easier to establish a relationship than to measure it. The relative risk of a disease in a user over a non-user is often the most difficult and

Table 1 Risks and benefits of oral contraceptive use

Beneficial		*Adverse*
Immediate	Reduced risk pelvic inflammatory disease	Increased risk myocardial infarction
	Reduced risk ectopic pregnancy	Increased risk stroke
Delayed	Reduced risk ovarian cancer	
	Reduced risk endometrial cancer	

least accurate measurement. In setting up FHI's equations the most pessimistic interpretation of relative risks has been accepted. For example, national statistics on deaths from cardio-vascular disease in Western countries show deaths to women of fertile age have *declined* substantially and consistently, during the years of greatest pill use. In order to allow for an increased relative risk of 3.0–5.0 suggested by the United Kingdom case-control studies, *non* pill-users would have had to have undergone a revolution in good health — a decline of 76–79% in deaths to women *not* using pills would have had to occur over an interval of twenty-four years. Nevertheless, the FHI model adopts the most cautious approach possible, using the high relative risks found in case-control data in its equations rather than the lower levels vital statistics would suggest (Table 2).

The model (Figure 2) shows that a woman below the age of thirty who takes oral contraceptives continuously for a five-year interval actually *increases* her expectation of life by a tiny, but calculable amount. A Western woman who takes the pill for five years and is over the age of thirty reduces her expectation of life, also by a small but measurable amount. Unfortunately, the data do not permit the separate calculation of risks by smokers and non-smokers, although what we know of the scale of interaction between smoking and oral contraceptives strongly suggests that, in non-smokers, the benefits of the pill might extend to all age groups up to age forty.

Table 2 Expectation of life and oral contraceptives

Side-effect	Relative risk	
Pelvic inflammatory disease	0.5	
Ovarian cancer	0.5	
Endometrial cancer	0.5	
Cervical cancer	1.5	
Myocardial infarction	3.0	(Age 30–39)
	4.0	(Age 40–49)
Stroke	5.0	(Age 30+)

In absolute terms, the maximum increase in life is an average of twelve days per pill-user and the maximum decrease eighty-eight days. For comparison, the woman who smokes a pack of cigarettes a day will reduce her expectation of life by 4.6 years. From the point of view of a woman's choice, or a physician's prescribing practice, pill use indubitably changes the profile of diseases to which a woman is exposed, but in everyday terms the risks and benefits of use virtually cancel one another out.

In the developed world less than 1% of deaths to adult women are pregnancy-related. In the developing world deaths due to pregnancy, childbirth and abortion account for 20–25% of deaths to adult women. When maternal mortality is fed into the overall equation of oral contraceptive risks and benefits over a lifetime then a woman in the developing world gains the greatest advantage. More women die from pregnancy in the Indian subcontinent in one *month* than die from the same causes in the United States, Canada, Western Europe, Eastern Europe, Japan, Australia and New Zealand in one *year*.

Yet it is one of the many paradoxes of pill use that the Indian government has consistently refused to make oral contraceptives available in any realistic way to the 100 million or more Indian women who

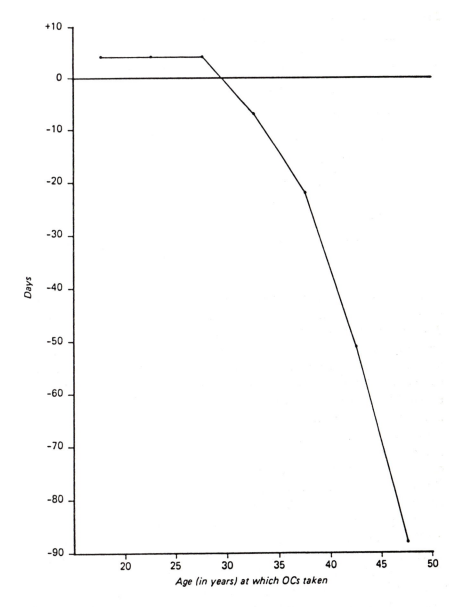

Figure 2 Change in life expectancy attributable to five years of oral contraception in the years specified: United States, 1978

live in the rural areas of that country. A decision to permit traditional practitioners to distribute pills could save thousands of lives from death in childbirth. When this was pointed out to a senior family planning leader in the country some years ago, she merely remarked, 'Ah, but those are natural deaths.'

The greatly reduced risk of pregnancy and labour to mother and child has been one of the undisputed triumphs of Western medicine in the last few decades. In England and Wales in 1950 there were 281 deaths due to complications of pregnancy, childbirth and abortion, while in 1975 there were only nineteen such deaths. The carnage of maternal deaths in the developing world continues at an unacceptably high level. If all the maternal deaths taking place in Third World countries were to occur at one place and at one time there would be an upsurge of humanitarian concern, but because maternal deaths are isolated, asynchronous events, they tend to go unnoticed: deaths due to childbirth at a global level are equivalent to crashing a jumbo jet full of pregnant and parturient women every five hours!

The provision of family planning is often the first element of primary health care that can be made available and the provision of pills and condoms would do a great deal to reduce the current wastage of adult and infant life. One-third of all the pregnancies in the world at the present moment are not wanted and most of these occur to older women of high parity who are at greatest risk of death and injury in childbirth. In Egypt, for example, a woman over thirty-five years of age having her first delivery is more than three times as likely to suffer perinatal loss as a woman aged nineteen to thirty-five after her first pregnancy. In a survey of twenty-nine developing countries it was found that if all deliveries could be spaced a minimum of two years, as is naturally the case among hunter-gatherer communities, then infant mortality would decline by half a million deaths per annum, even in the absence of any other improvements in health care. Not only do many women die because they lack skilled care in pregnancy at childbirth, but very large numbers suffer life-long injuries. Prolonged obstructed labour can lead to death of the tissues separating the vagina from the bladder or rectum, giving rise to permanent urinary or fecal incontinence and turning the unfortunate victim into a foul-smelling outcast in her own community.

Calculations based on expectation of life are necessarily contrived. They permit comparison of existing and any possible new epidemiology, but the lack of perspective surrounding pill use goes much deeper than a failure to comprehend the limitations of epidemiology, or accurately to read the implication of the relative risks that have been measured.

In 1985 the American College of Obstetricians and Gynecologists sponsored a Gullup poll on American attitudes towards contraception. Three-quarters of American women and 62% of men believe there are 'substantial risks in using the birth control pill'. A risk of cancer is at the top of most people's list despite the fact the pill seems to reduce the risk of two important reproductive cancers. When asked to compare the risks of using the pill to childbearing, 46% of American women thought it was more risky. In fact, childbearing is twice as dangerous as the risk of cardio-vascular disease among oral contraceptive users and over ten times as dangerous as pill use by non-smokers under age thirty-five. In 1985/86 FHI and the International Health Foundation (IHF) conducted a survey of consumer perceptions in sixteen countries worldwide from Britain and Italy to Senegal and Indonesia. Everywhere the same picture of pessimism, gross misunderstanding and profound misinformation exists. Women believe the pill is reliable and easy to use but regard it as extremely dangerous. As in the USA, so in Thailand, Sri Lanka, Mexico, Costa Rica and Chile the pill is falsely perceived as more dangerous than pregnancy even though in developing countries the actual ratio of pregnancies to oral contraceptive risks, as has been emphasised, is substantially more in favour of the pill. Unfounded assertions that hormonal contraceptives cause subsequent infertility and, if the woman does get pregnant, congenital abnormalities, are even more common outside the USA. Exceptionally few women surveyed know the pill protects against ovarian and uterine cancer and pelvic inflammatory disease. Cancer phobia in relation to the pill is widespread in developed and developing countries, including, for example, a myth in Chile that the pill causes stomach cancer. Why do pill consumers from West Germany to Nigeria have similar perceptions and why are there the same pessimistic misunderstandings from San Francisco to Ujung Pandang?

Firstly, the pill is still regarded as a prescription drug and the fact that women are examined before it is given has probably helped to establish an aura of danger. It is interesting that in the Philippines, where oral contraceptives are available over the counter, women are less pessimistic than in some other countries. In reality the two most important contra-indications to use — age over forty and smoking in a woman over thirty-five — depend on the history of the user, not on physical examination. Users do not understand that the physician's examination is largely an opportunity for preventive medicine, providing an occasion to take the blood pressure, do a cervical smear and examine the breasts.

Secondly, manufacturers themselves may have unwittingly contributed to undermining their own product. It is easy to forget that the pharmaceutical industry has never sold a packet of pills to a woman. All their advertising has thus of necessity been focused on the prescribing physician, and in promoting their products they have needed to emphasise such things as blood clotting in order to claim their brand is less dangerous than a competitor's.

Thirdly, those groups who are morally opposed to artificial contraception go to great lengths to exaggerate any risks that exist. In the 1920s and 1930s, barrier vaginal methods of contraception, such as the diaphragm and condom, were subject to the same hostility. Today, neither a user nor a physician would seriously hold that barrier methods cause cancer, but a generation ago some prominent gynecologists were only too ready to make such an assertion.

Finally, and most important of all, the pill is intimately linked with sex, and that is an area where we are all insecure. Studies have been performed on how people evaluate everyday risks. On the whole, people underestimate the significance of common day-to-day risks such as, for example, the risk of infant death from measles but overestimate dramatic and well publicised risks.

The fact that the pill risks are being widely publicised in the press and that it has something to do with sex seems to set up an environment where risks are exaggerated and misunderstood. The old song,

'It's Immoral, It's Illegal or It Makes You Fat', might be aptly applied to fertility regulation.

The pill forces us to think about the world in many new ways. Over the past decade a vision of human reproductive mortality has arisen which takes into account a lifelong perspective of the risks associated with pregnancy and childbirth, with the means to control fertility such as deaths from abortion and oral contraceptive use.

Maternal mortality has fallen because of better health and obstetric care and because yesterday's older, high parity women, who were at greatest risk for death during pregnancy or delivery, today practise voluntary family planning. The precipitous fall in maternal mortality and concomitant rise in fertility regulation have created a situation where the absolute number of deaths due to pregnancy and child-birth, in countries such as Britain or America, is now of the same order of magnitude as deaths due to the regulation of fertility (oral contraceptives, induced abortion, IUD and voluntary sterilisation deaths.

In passing it is important to notice that with modern patterns of childbearing a woman spends many more years using birth control than she does being pregnant or giving birth and the risks per unit of exposure are correspondingly smaller for contraceptives than for pregnancy.

Deaths due to pregnancy and due to fertility regulation are inextricably related. Over the past thirty years deaths due to both categories have seen a marked reduction. It is important to remember that if women are to go on benefiting from insights into reproductive health then attention must continue to be focused both on further improvements in obstetrics *and* on a better understanding of the risks associated with fertility regulation. The legislation of abortion has led to a dramatic reduction in deaths from this method of birth control.

The greater part of the deaths related to contraception are cardio-vascular deaths due to oral contraceptive use rather than mortality related to IUDs. The decline in death rates due to this cause between 1975 and 1982 reflects a better screening and counselling of women at risk for oral contraceptive use. The American College of Obstetricians and Gynecologists estimates that currently there are about five deaths per year for every 100 000 pill-users. But if no pill-user smoked and if no one over the age of thirty-five used oral contraceptives, then this rate would drop to 0.7 deaths for each 100 000 pill-users. This compares to about ten maternal deaths for every 100 000 births in the USA.

Women have and always will carry most of the risks associated with reproduction, but coitus itself, like most good things in life, also carries a measurable chance of death, and a not insignificant number of cardio-vascular accidents and coronary thrombosis to men, as well as women, occur during sexual intercourse. As one bumper sticker proclaims, 'Living is hazardous to health!'.

In addition to those deaths directly related to pregnancy and its control, there is a less obvious, but numerically more significant, mortality related to patterns of childbearing over a reproductive lifetime. It is this vision of women's health which oral contraceptives illuminate in a particularly exciting way, yet it remains the least understood aspect of oral contraceptive use within both the medical and lay communities.

Epidemiology points out statistical relationships; it is up to the biologist to provide an exegesis on epidemiological findings. The biologist sees us as a mammal subjected to the special stresses of civilised living. Modern living, by lowering the age of puberty and altering patterns of breastfeeding and reducing infant mortality, has made contraception a necessity. But there is also another set of biological patterns in the background which are uniquely relevant to oral contraceptives.

In the present world, women frequently delay childbearing into their twenties, have few children and rarely breastfeed for more than a few months. Thus, they may have 350 menstrual cycles in a lifetime. This change carries with it a series of pathologies. Endometriosis and fibromyomata are partially linked to delayed and infrequent childbearing and there is a strong and consistent correlation between a woman's pattern of childbearing and breast, ovarian and uterine cancer. Breast cancer attacks one in eleven American women and kills one in eighteen; ovarian cancer is often well advanced and incurable at the time of diagnosis.

Epidemiological studies of populations of Japanese who have emigrated to the United States and then had children demonstrate that the incidence of breast cancer changes in these two generations from the low level found in Japan to the high level found in the United States: thus, reproductive cancers, like lung cancer, appear in part to be a result of environmental changes. Breast, ovarian and endometrial cancers have all been shown to be more common in women who are exposed to long, uninterrupted intervals of repeated ovulation.

Among many lay people, as well as some members of the medical profession, the perception has grown that the use of hormonal contraceptives is 'unnatural'. It is perhaps more realistic to appreciate that modern living makes a great many unnatural demands on the reproductive system of women, certain of which have serious and demonstrably harmful effects.

The fact that oral contraceptive use, if sustained for several years, should approximately halve the risk of ovarian and uterine cancer makes good biological sense. The fact that repeated and large-scale studies of breast cancer have shown no conclusive relationship with oral contraceptive use remains a puzzle. Breast cancer affects more women than any other cancer. The human breast is exquisitely sensitive to ovarian hormones and breast cancer itself is influenced by a woman's history of childbearing and often responds to changes in the hormone environment. It would be very surprising if the steroids in the contraceptive pill did not affect patterns of breast cancer in the same way as they do other reproductive cancers. However, it is also possible that the pill could have different effects if taken at different times in a woman's life, that different pills could act in different ways and that the pill could have a different effect on the initiation of cancer or on the progress of already established cancers. In the latter case, there is some evidence to suggest that if a woman is unfortunate enough to develop breast cancer it spreads more slowly if she is on the pill at the time the disease is first diagnosed. On top of these complications, breast cancer itself is not a homogeneous disease and pills could have different effects on different types of breast cancer.

Breast cancer is more common in women who bear their first child late in life. It is also more common in those who have an early menarche or a late menopause. It is less common in women who breastfeed their children. In short, purposeless ovarian cycles appear to predispose the breast to malignancy.

Now there is considerable evidence that oral contraceptives reduce ovarian and endometrial cancer. It is reasonable to ask if the pill may also be protective against breast cancer. Unfortunately, this does not seem to be the case. Several large trials have compared breast cancer among pill-users and non-users and overall they have shown no difference whatsoever in the incidence of the disease between those using oral contraceptives and controlled groups. In view of what we know about breast cancer this is a surprising result.

The commonness of the disease and the complexities of the hormonal environment in which it develops make it necessary to look at subgroups of women taking the pill. Epidemiologists have begun to do this but the results are mysterious and conflicting. Some studies have suggested there is a rise in the instance of breast cancer among women who take the pill under the age of 25 and/or take it before their first pregnancy. However, these findings have been contradicted by other equally well conducted studies. It is possible that the overall apparent lack of relationship between oral contraceptive use and breast cancer conceals groups of women where the pill has an adverse effect and groups of women where it has a protective effect.

Not only is the epidemiology difficult to do but the breast is a difficult organ to study. Unlike the cervix, the key cellular changes which take place during the ovarian cycle and pregnancy cannot be monitored. Biopsies are possible but only ethically acceptable if there is a suspicion of disease and not out of biological curiosity.

Data are emerging to suggest that the pattern of cellular proliferation during the normal menstrual cycle differs from that of the endometrium, therefore the progestational content of oral contraceptives could be influential on the possible development of breast cancer. Human beings are the only animals where the breast arises at puberty and there is no adequate animal model to help us predict the effect of hormones on breast disease. In the rat, the interesting observation has been made that a single shot of Depo-Provera early in fertile life has the same effect as pregnancy and protects the breast against cancer later on. Although the species differences are great it is possible that artificial hormones could be manipulated in such a way as to markedly reduce a woman's risk of breast cancer late in life.

(In Britain and the USA a woman's lifetime risk of death from childbirth is approximately 1 in 5000. Her risk of dying of breast cancer is 1 in 20 or more. This suggests that while we are judging steroidal contraceptives on their efficacy and side-effects we should try to develop mechanisms for judging them by their potential effect on the human breast and subsequent risk of cancer. A small increase in the risk of breast cancer due to some unfortunate combination of effects of the current pills in a subgroup of women would be a very serious finding. A combination of steroids tailored to protect the teenage breast against the risk of cancer at the menopause and later, in the same way as a first pregnancy protects the breast, would be one of the miracles of the 20th century. Much more thought and effort need to be put into the fulfilment of this vision of reproductive health.

It would be over simple to suggest that today's steroidal contraceptives meet the twin goals of contraception in ensuring a healthy body at the menopause, free of cancer and other pathologies related to lifelong patterns of childbearing, but it is reasonable to suggest that the pill has proved the first halting step in this direction. Certainly, physicians and medical scientists would be wise to set the goal of developing methods of contraception which are not only simple, reversible and have a minimum of harmful effects but which also forestall the pathologies associated with late childbearing and non-pregnancy. It is possible that in 100, or even 500, years' time women may still be using a systemically active method of contraception at least for some part of their reproductive lives and probably in the teens and twenties, both to prevent pregnancy and to mimic those changes in the lifelong pattern of reproduction associated with protection against breast cancer and other forms of reproductive pathology which occur when pregnancy is delayed or never takes place at all. To delay childbearing by the use of a condom or periodic abstinence is more unnatural than using hormonal contraceptives.

Epidemiologists deal in probabilities; biologists can always ask more questions than they can provide answers; but administrators, like individuals deciding on contraceptive methods, must make 'yes' or 'no' decisions. They must react not only to real and perceived physical risks of fertility regulation methods, but also to political and logistic side-effects. Ultimately, all administrative decisions balancing risks and benefits boil down to empirical human judgments.

Nowhere is this truer than in the field of contraception. The pill is still not licensed as a contraceptive in Japan, but is promoted by street advertisements in Korea; somebody is wrong. In Thailand pills are distributed by villagers with one day's training, in India they are supposed to be on prescription; somebody is wrong. Common sense, experience and epidemiological observation support simple distribution systems. In 1973, the International Planned Parenthood Federation's central medical committee concluded that 'the limitation of all contraceptive distribution to doctors' prescriptions makes the method geographically, economically, sometimes culturally inaccessible to many women.' In 1976, a Joint Working Party on Oral Contraceptives set up by the Department of Health and Social Security in Britain stated[3], 'We do not regard it as necessary to restrict authority to issue prescriptions for oral contraceptives to doctors.'

Logically, the need for medical prescription turns on four questions:

1. Is the drug addictive?
2. Does the dose have to be adjusted for each individual?
3. Is overdose lethal?
4. Are there certain categories of people for whom the drug is especially dangerous?

In relation to the pill, the answer to the first three questions is 'No' and known risk groups are mainly categorised on the patient's history and not the results of physical examination. Doctors can safely and responsibly delegate the distribution of the pill to lay workers. An FHI sponsored study in Matamuros, Mexico, compared those receiving pills through medical channels and those buying them over-the-counter and examined and tested all groups for diseases such as hypertension and diabetes. On the one hand, physicians did not follow the textbook and on the other women with chronic diseases excluded themselves from oral contraceptives, even though objective examination showed it would have been reasonable for the women to use the method. In fact, more women did not use the pill who could have done so than did use the method and should not have done so.

Decisions about delegation must not be confused with statements about the absence or presence of side-effects. A community-based distribution programme acknowledges that there are risks associated with oral contraceptive use, but in nearly all cases experience has shown that lay people and auxiliaries can work together with the available specialist skills in such a way as to provide not only a broad service but also one with the optimum level of care. Objective analysis shows that medical practitioners are not always the most consistent supervisors of fertility regulation methods[1]. Most methods are so simple that doctors find it difficult to maintain a high level of interest; the non-specialists may do a routine task better than the specialist; an auxiliary may perform as well as a doctor.

In the last analysis, the opinion of all the specialists and administrators is secondary to what goes on in the mind of a woman taking her first pill. Epidemiologists have not conducted a careful random trial comparing the relative risks of purchasing the pill without prescription and of having an abortion with a bent coathanger, although these are real choices for many millions of women. The biologist has not found a way of quantitating the cerebral emotions associated with attempting to bring up five children with love and dignity on a few dollars a day, compared with the risk of cardio-vascular disease on the pill, although this is what we are talking about in India. The committee of medical administrators, who sit in an air-conditioned office of a capital city deciding what tasks should be delegated to medical auxiliaries, cannot know what it means to be in labour for four days, attended by a traditional midwife, to be delivered of a dead baby and left with a rectovaginal fistula.

Individuals make daily domestic decisions about their own families and themselves. Persons seeking contraceptive advice are usually healthy, unconcerned about the demographic problems of their country, but motivated by a desire to provide the best for their children and a wish to enjoy the pleasures and satisfaction of sexual intercourse with their partner. The individual perspective can easily come into conflict with that of the physicians or administrators. In reality, fertility regulation differs philosophically from other branches of medicine. Individuals make their own diagnosis: 'I suspect I am fertile; I know I am having regular intercourse; I have decided not to have a child.' The physician is meeting people's choices, not diagnosing and treating their diseases. Some doctors accept this element of service, but others find it a disturbing challenge.

For the individual, (the voluntary control of fertility enhances the quality of human reproduction by helping to confine pregnancy to those years in a woman's life when she is least at risk of mortality and morbidity by enabling her to provide maximum security for her offspring and by adding to the emotional aspects of sex for both partners.) How should an individual use the insights of the biologist and the epidemiologist to assign values to the risks and benefits of fertility control, and what should he or she expect from medical advisors?

The perspective of the individual user is the most important — but also the most difficult to establish. The individual contemplating the use of contraceptives will almost certainly rate sexual activity as more important than most other domestic pleasure pursuits. The statistics of the unusual are easy to pervert, yet illustrations of the level of certain daily risks demonstrate how the dangers of contraception, because of their sexual links, become more widely publicised than those of some other choices made by individuals. The risk of death from drowning for American adolescents is 11.7 per 100 000, and for men aged 20–24 it is 7.6 per 100 000. There is many more times the likelihood of death in the family if the father has an outboard motor-boat than if the mother takes the pill; there is as much chance of death from one hour in a sailplane (4.4 deaths per 1000 hours) than from one year of pill using. In the USA, there is a greater danger from the *accidental* use of firearms (2.5 deaths per 100 000 of the population) than from the use of the pill by a non-smoker. Between 1963 and 1973 approximately 50 000 Americans were killed fighting in Vietnam and during the same interval nearly 85 000 were killed at home in the USA with hand-guns. A male born into a big US city has a one in thirty-three chance of being murdered, while a US serviceman, during the Second World War, had a one in fifty chance of being killed. A young black male (25-35) in the USA has about 100 times the chance of being murdered than his wife or girlfriend has of dying from use of the pill[4]. It does seem paradoxical that the US government spends over 200 million dollars a year controlling the introduction of drugs, but is unable to legislate against hand-guns.

Almost without exception, oral contraceptives contribute to individual health and to the well-being of the community. One measurable impact of the introduction of oral contraceptives is that between 1965 and 1970 the mean coital frequency among women in the US who are married and living with their husbands increased by almost 25%[4].

One useful way of describing specific risks to life is to suppose that all causes of death could be removed, except for the risk under discussion (Table 3). For every woman who dies as a result of oral contraceptives in Britain, many hundred men and women die because they smoke. The annual mortality for cigarette-induced lung cancer in Britain is 90 per 100 000, and for heavy smokers (who retain the cigarette in their mouths between puffs) 410 per 100 000. Cigarettes present the foremost preventable cause of death in the United States. 'For the American male (and probably likewise for the female) aged 40–79 who smokes a pack or more cigarettes per day, smoking is an environmental hazard equal to all other hazards to life combined.'[5]

An element in the poker game which decides the availability of drugs is the right of individuals to take risks with their lives. On the whole, we apply more stringent rules to the risks that other people take than we do to ourselves.

The individual may be alarmed by the newspaper headlines of young women who die on the pill and be unable to place them in epidemiological perspective. But, in her own decision-making, other factors also come into play. The personal and economic consequences of one more child are usually significant to the individual woman, while the mortality associated with pregnancy may be discounted as a significant risk. If the balancing of risks does occur to the individual,

Table 3 How long would a person live if they had only one risk of death? (US and UK data)

Risk	Life expectancy (years)
Smoking 40 cigarettes per day	100
Riding a motorcycle 10 h per week	300
Drinking a bottle of wine per day	1 300
Driving a car 10 h per week	3 500
Power boating once a month	6 000
Having a baby every year	10 000
Playing football twice a week	25 000
Staying home for 200 h per year watching television (man aged 16–68)	50 000
Using oral contraceptives (non smoker)*	63 000
Travelling by train 100 h per year	200 000
Using an IUD	200 000
Being struck by lightning	10 000 000
Being hit by a falling aeroplane	50 000 000

* The calculation only considers cardio-vascular risks and omits the benefits of the pill, such as reduced ovarian cancer. The risks of other steroidal contraceptives, such as injectable Depo-Provera, are omitted. To date, no human deaths have been associated with these drugs and, as of the present, they would have to be associated with a separate category of 'immortality' in this table. (Adapted from Rochat, R. and Hatcher, R.)

it is in relation to the question 'Am I going to be pregnant this month?' and not based on a cumulative lifetime hazard. The individual making a contraceptive choice is rarely looking at public health outcomes and will arrive at different conclusions from the epidemiologist. The individual is facing a tree with branching choices, not an equation with balancing statistics. The millions of women around the world whom studies show believe the pill is so dangerous might be more comfortable if they understood that the absolute risk to life of oral contraceptive use is *probably less than smoking one cigarette a day*. And now we know that for most groups life-saving benefits equal or outweigh demonstrable hazards, the adage that cigarettes should be on prescription and pills in vending machines seems appropriate.

While the perceived health benefits and hazards of oral contraceptives have been widely publicised, the pill's impact on society and on family life has been discussed even more passionately. To some, it seems the pill was the engine of change in the sexual revolution; to others, it appears as no more than a symbol. Certainly, at a global level oral contraceptives have reached a high prevalence of use in societies with very different sexual mores. Few communities could be as different as the United States of America and the People's Republic of China: one is capitalist and a higher percentage of its citizens attend church each Sunday than in any other industrialised nation; the other has a communist, atheist government; in China prostitution has been virtually eliminated, premarital sexual intercourse is unusual, society goes to great lengths to counsel couples with stormy marriages to remain together and even masturbation is regarded with Victorian prudery as something intrinsically harmful; in the United States prostitution is visible in any large city and legal in at least one state, premarital sex is the rule and there is an epidemic of teenage pregnancies. The mean duration of married life for a couple without children is a mere five years, sex is openly discussed on radio and television and everything from automobiles to ocean cruises is promoted by scantily clad, provocative pictures of young women. Yet in both countries oral contraceptives have been widely used and it would seem unlikely that they could be a major driving force in the sexual behaviour of society on one side of the Pacific and yet be irrelevant on the other.

From a public health point of view, there has been a marked rise in the prevalence of sexually transmitted diseases in most Western industrial societies since World War II. However, when the figures are plotted out in detail it is seen that the climb in venereal diseases began before the rise in oral contraceptive use (Figure 3). It is the clinical experience of those who have counselled unmarried girls in Western societies that only, literally, one in a thousand young women seeks a prescription of oral contraceptives while she is still a virgin. The vast majority begin intercourse and often have some kind of pregnancy scare, or, tragically, actually conceive before they choose to use oral contraceptives. Having said this, there is a marked difference in social

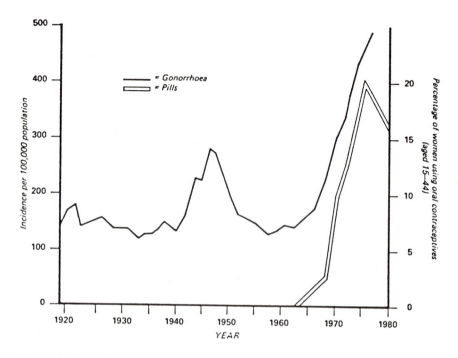

Figure 3 Sexually transmitted diseases under oral contraceptive use, in the United Kingdom

attitudes toward the availability of the pill for young people in various Western countries. In the Netherlands the pill is widely available and it is expected that responsible young people will seek contraceptive protection when they begin to have intercourse. In the United States, attitudes are ambivalent and as a consequence, while the prevalence of sexual intercourse by age nineteen is similar in the Netherlands and the USA, the use of contraceptives (and of the pill in particular) is considerably lower in the USA than in Holland and the pregnancy rate is approximately seven times as high.

In the 1960s the pill presented the greatest single challenge to Roman Catholic couples and Roman Catholic theologians. John Rock, the only gynecologist on the pill's inventing triumvirate, was himself a lifelong, devout Roman Catholic. In 1963 he wrote *The Time Has Come: A Catholic Doctor's Proposal to End the Battle Over Birth Control*[6]. With customary sincerity he told the story how vividly he remembered the advice given to him by the family priest, Father Finnick, when he was a young fourteen-year-old: 'John, always stick to your conscience. Never let anyone else keep it for you — and I mean *anyone* else.' Rock argued that the pill, like pregnancy, mimicked the natural and theologically acceptable control of fertility: 'My reasoning is based, in part, on the fact that the rhythm method, which is sanctioned by the Church, depends precisely on the secretion of progesterone from the ovaries, which action these compounds (the pill) merely duplicate... These organs supply progesterone at those times when nature seeks to protect a fertilised ovum, from jeopardy. Since the intellect is also part of a woman's natural being, it too is charged with the duty of protection against potential danger.'

A year later, in Britain Anne Biezanek[7], a young Roman Catholic, woman doctor with seven children, wrote a much more empassioned plea for the use of oral contraceptives, called *All Things New*. A theological scholarship in philosophy explicitly derived from natural law seemed ready to evolve thoughtfully and with reverence for older traditions, just as the same Church had initially rejected but then come to live with usury, or the heliocentric interpretation of the solar system. In 1966 Pope Paul VI assembled a Commission for the Study of Population and Family Life. It consisted of a group of clerics led by Cardinal Ottaviani and eventually involved sixty-four theologians, physicians, demographers and family counsellors. Overall the Commission voted sixty to four for changes in the Church's teaching towards contraception, and the pill in particular. The Cardinals are thought to have voted nine to six in favour of contraception. The first ten years after the invention of the pill had seen cerebrate theological justifications for change. The most significant event in this decade of ferment was Pope John XXIII's Vatican Council II, launched in 1962. The summary document from the Council (*Gaudium et Spes*) carefully avoided the age-old insistence that the *primary* purpose of marriage was the procreation of children. Instead, it elevated the conjugal expression of love as a self-justifying purpose of marriage and it explicitly assured parents that they alone had the right to decide on the spacing of their children, although they were exhorted to make their decisions after solemn thought and to 'consult the interests of the family group, of temporal society, and of the Church itself'.

The great majority of Church members endorsed the responsible use of oral contraceptives and millions of women, with every reason to expect Vatican approval, happily swallowed the near magic pill each night. Pope Paul VI's Encyclical, *Humanae Vitae*, was published in July 1968. In it the Pope concluded: 'Whoever deliberately renders coitus sterile attacks its meaning as an expression of mutual self-giving.' Around the world there was astonishment and in at least one city the Papal Nuncio could not believe what he was reading. Within forty-eight hours a group of American theologians, based at a Catholic university in Washington, challenged the Encyclical. Before the debate was over 600 Catholic scholars made clear their disagreement with the Pope. They pointed out that while the Pope insisted that every coital act must be 'open to the transmission of life', biologically this was just not possible and therefore the morality of human sex had to be judged on the commitment of the couple themselves. In Europe many Episcopates filtered the Encyclical to their flock with subtle alterations: contraceptives might be 'a disorder' but not necessarily 'a sin'. John Rock's plea for the primacy of the human conscience was reiterated.

The body of the Church continued to move further and further away from the Vatican's teaching. In the early 1960s non-Catholic families had an average of just over three children and Catholic families of just over four. By the mid-1970s the fertility of the two groups was identical at just over two children. In 1965, 59% of Catholics were using a contraceptive and 70% of non-Catholics, but in ten years the use in both groups rose and the gap was closed to a mere three percentage point difference. In 1965, 50% more non-Catholics than Catholics were using oral contraceptives but by 1975 use was identical at 34% of all women in both categories[8].

The trauma the little pill caused the Church was as great as that of Martin Luther's twenty-three theses. Before the widespread use of the pill, in the early 1960s, 70% of Catholics attended the Mass weekly but by the mid–1970s only 44% were doing so. A National Opinion Research Center Poll conducted in 1977 found that only 4% of Catholics in their twenties believed contraception was wrong. Young people were especially deeply troubled and whereas 80% had been attending Mass weekly in 1963 only 13% did so in 1979. Vast numbers of priests and nuns left clerical orders, in the largest single number of cases because they could not accept the Church's teaching on birth control.

The tragedy of *Humanae Vitae* is that it came so close to escaping from the narrow perspectives of the early Fathers of the Church who saw human coitus as analogous to that of a cat or a donkey and solely for procreation. Indeed, Pope Paul VI explicitly called for a total biological and Christian vision of human reproduction in *Humanae Vitae*. Sadly, the lifelong perspective of reproduction which biologists were able to provide and the vision of the whole human being, which theologians sought, never came together. *Humanae Vitae* ended up teaching that human beings were rabbits, in the sense that every act of sex had to have the associated possibility of pregnancy. At a practical level, the world–wide network of parish priests, many living under harsh conditions and in close contact with communities struggling to achieve economic dignity in the Third World, were turned back from the mission they might have conducted of using the human intellect to help our species adjust to the complex conditions of a modern world.

Clinically, a medicine that adds a tiny but demonstrable time to the expectation of life has accumulated a reputation of extreme hazard. Socially, the pill has been accused of initiating a sexual revolution which preceded its availability. As with Galileo, the Church misjudged the scientific and human integrity of an immensely important discovery. Faced with the threat of the Inquisition, Galileo murmured under his breath, 'It still moves'; John Rock proclaimed to the world, 'Always stick to your conscience'.

REFERENCES

1. The Boston Women's Health Book Collective. *The New Our Bodies Our Selves*. Simon & Schuster, New York

2. Department of Health and Social Security (1976). *Report of the Joint Working Group on Oral Contraceptives*. Her Majesty's Stationary Office, London
3. Peel, J. and Potts, M. (1969). *Textbook of Contraceptive Practice*. Cambridge University Press, Cambridge, England
4. Potts, M, Speidel, J. J. and Kessel, E. (1978). Relative risks of various means of fertility control used in less developed countries. In Sciarra, J., Zatuchni, G. I. and Speidel, J. J. (eds) *Risks, Benefits, and Controversies in Fertility Control*, p. 28. Harper & Row, Hagerstown, MD
5. Rock, J. (1963). *The Time Has Come*. Longman, London
6. Biezanek, A. (1964). *All Things New*. Pan Books, London
7. Murphy, F. X. (1981). *Catholic Perspectives on Population Issues*. Population Reference Bureau
8. Cartwright, A. (1970). *Parents and Family Planning Services*. Rutledge & Kegan Paul, London
9. MacMahon, B., Cole, P. and Brauns, T. (1973). Etiology of human breast cancer: a review. *J. Natl. Cancer Inst.*, **50**, 21
10. Ravenholt, R. T. (1978). Cigarette smoking: magnitude of the hazard. Paper presented at the Annual Meeting of the Epidemic Intelligence Service, Center for Disease Control, Atlanta, GA
11. Smith, M. and Kane, P. (1975). *The Pill Off Prescription*. Birth Control Trust, London

Chapter 10

The Pill and the Future

'The ability to control one's own fertility now gives to each individual woman a degree of freedom and choice greater than is provided by any other aspect of health care.' Potts and Diggory in 1983 made this claim, summarising the developments in contraception over the previous fifty years, and concluded, perhaps more controversially, that on a global scale 'the right of access to contraception may be even more important than the right of access to the ballot box'.

In almost only a quarter of a century the role of women in modern society had undergone a revolution, due to the effective and reliable contraception that the pill had brought them. What therefore of the future? Is it likely that as dramatic a change as that brought about by Russell Marker's discovery of how to synthesise steroid hormones from a vegetable in the 1940s will occur again with some other pharmaceutical innovation? Will there be, around the corner, the comparatively modest liberation from the necessity of having to swallow a pill each night for the woman of tomorrow? Will some entirely different agent usable for the effective control of fertility be discovered which perhaps involves the male, who after all equally shares the responsibility for each pregnancy conceived? Is there anything waiting to be discovered that is absolutely safe and free from any possible or unwanted side-effect? Carl Djerassi wrote at the end of his book *The Politics of Contraception*: 'Of the money now being spent on new contraceptive development, essentially none is being allocated to developing new chemical entities suitable for ovulation inhibition by the progestational hormone mechanism. Therefore the next hormonal pill for women — if there is going to be a next — is unlikely to be a steroid.'

Egon Diczfalusy, however, of the World Health Organisation, recognising the astronomic costs now facing pharmaceutical companies in the development of any new agent and the satisfaction of the requirements of the drug regulatory authorities asks: 'With present day estimates ranging from 30 to 70 million dollars, can multiple investments of this order of magnitude ever be recovered by industry for the development of improved fertility regulating drugs to be used mainly in developing countries? The answer is, probably not.' Yet the Vice Premier of the Chinese Peoples' Republic, Chen Mu-Hua, speaking on behalf of nearly a quarter of the world's population has said: 'Our people are dissatisfied, and demand better methods, and we have to meet this demand.'

When a woman buys one month's supply of oral contraceptives in a pharmacy in the USA she pays between $12 and $18. The same product in the same package made by the same manufacturer can be bought in bulk for International Family Planning Programmes for literally one hundredth the price. A very large part of this extraordinary difference is money set aside for the issues of product liability. Any manufacturer of oral contraceptives in the United States has to expect a continual series of court cases coming up, many of which he will lose. The cases related to the pill are sometimes based on good scientific evidence and compensation is given to women who have genuinely suffered a rare but serious adverse effect. Other cases, which perhaps represent little more than the fertile imagination of lawyers, may also be found in favour of the plaintiff.

The volume of oral contraceptive use and their long history of legal cases allow the manufacturers to set aside sufficient funds to deal with product liability cases. However, they remain reluctant to introduce new methods of contraception, including new formulations of contraceptive steroids, because in the absence of such experience it is virtually impossible to guess the level of product liability cases that are likely to arise in the USA. Product liability has ousted intrauterine devices off the market (even though some remain FDA approved) and has threatened the sale of spermicides.

The dilemma of the future is therefore between the needs, convenience, and safety requirements of the developed world and the price of achieving them, and the needs, convenience and accessibility, as well as the safety of the population of the developing countries and whether they can afford it. As things are today, there is little hope of a compromise, beyond some modest refinements of the pharmaceutical agents used in the last three decades, to ameliorate their biological impact and yet maintain contraceptive effectiveness. Attitudes towards fertility control have so changed that sexually active people world-wide now feel that they have a right to the perfect contraceptive: effective, simple, reversible and free from unwanted side-effects. They are often frustrated and invariably nonplussed to find that it still does not exist.

THE MALE PILL

Physiologically there are more sites where reproduction can be interrupted in the male than in the female but there are also more profound biological problems. Men produce sperm throughout their adult lives and there is no natural way for turning off fertility in the way that pregnancy prevents further ovulation in women.

There are a number of chemicals (e.g., nitrogen mustards and cytotoxic agents) which inhibit sperm production but they affect other cell growth in the male body and are variable in effectiveness and toxicity.

In the 1950s agents known as nitrofurans were assessed, but they produced intolerable nausea. Another agent suppressed sperm production but severe and adverse reactions occurred whenever the user drank alcohol. The anti-androgen cyproterone-acetate has been tested as a male pill. This works by suppressing the function of the pituitary but it also suppresses other male hormone production and therefore directly alters male sexual impulse and desire. Testoterone can be administered by repeated injections at ten day intervals, to suppress sperm production, but in trials an escape of its effects was found, with fertile sperms appearing at 70–80 day intervals. Gossypol, or cotton seed oil, a poly-phenol substance, when used for cooking was observed to be associated with unintentional infertility in males, and testicular atrophy (shrinkage) in parts of China. This excited world-wide interest and investigation showed that it impaired the fructose utilisation (i.e., energy consumption for swimming) of the sperms, but severe depletion of body calcium levels was also found, rendering it dangerous and unacceptable for medical use.

Several other agents used in therapy of disease (e.g., beta-blockers for hypertension, and salazopyrin for colitis) have been found to produce partial suppression of sperm production, but their actions in doing this remain as yet relatively uninvestigated. It has also been suggested that spin-offs from experiments and research involved in the rapidly developing techniques and practice of *in-vitro* fertilisation (IVF, or 'test-tube' baby production) may reveal some ways in which sperm once produced may be rendered incapable of achieving fertilisation.

Nevertheless, so far the picture is best summarised by Potts (1983): 'While a male oral pill would be a considerable advance in family planning, given the current low levels of investment in contraceptive research and the biological complexity of interrupting male reproduction without the danger of producing abnormal sperm, *it seems unlikely that such a product will be widely used in the next 10–15 years, and perhaps not even before the twenty-first century.*'

THE 'ONCE A MONTH' OR 'MORNING AFTER' PILL

In the last ten years there has been ever-increasing research into the 'releasing' hormones derived via the hypothalamus of the brain, the ones that control the secretion levels of the steroid hormones from the other endocrine glands of the body: pituitary, thyroid and ovary. Ironically, much of the stimulus for this research has been derived from attempts to overcome infertility in women suffering from ovarian disease or hormonal aberrations that prevent ovulation, but then Rock and Pincus' earliest work in Boston with what ultimately became the pill was an attempt to treat the problem of infertility. Already, therefore, doses of the anti-luteinising hormone agent are being assessed for their capability of suppressing ovulation, and quantities as small as 50 microgram on three successive days in each cycle are demonstrating their potential as a contraceptive. It can be administered via a nasal spray but its reliability is as yet not fully assessed, and its cost is exorbitant — over US $300 a month.

Since the secretion of progesterone (from the corpus luteum or yellow body of the egg cell's follicle left behind on the ovary's surface) is essential for the survival of the embryo after implantation in the wall of the uterus, the investigation of anti-progesterone agents or inhibitors of progesterone secretion may offer another means of fertility control. However, such an agent is not a contraceptive, but is fundamentally an abortion-producing agent. Roussel (a French pharmaceutical firm) are currently investigating a synthetic anti-progesterone agent coded as 'RU 486', which is given for four days before menstruation is due or early in a known pregnancy. The results (reported in Berlin in October 1985 at the World Congress of Obstetricians and Gynecologists) gave some optimistic hope, but too many women remained pregnant or bled with a 'missed' abortion and had therefore to have surgical intervention with dilation and curretting of the uterus, for it to be considered, as yet, a success. It has the makings of a 'once a month' pill, but it is not made yet.

In the early 1970s prostaglandins were hailed as 'wonder drugs' in that they could 'bring on' a delayed menstrual period — in other words as abortion-producers. Some of the prostaglandin group have, in fact, proved useful when used as pessaries to induce labour in women in whom delivery of a baby is delayed or overdue. However, in securing an earlier evacuation of the uterus by stimulating uterine contractions their use has been disappointing. Although they were discovered as a group of chemical substances in 1935, by Von Euler in Sweden, and have been known for their effects for over fifty years, further research into their use and modification of their chemical structure has been relatively slow. Short-term side-effects and incomplete evacuation of the pregnant uterus (as with RU 486) have proved to be problems. 'Multinational corporations have become so frightened by possible litigation and by the hostility of a vocal minority that some have made an explicit decision *not* to conduct further trials on human volunteers,' claimed Potts (1983) in considering why the 'once a month' abortion pill had not been developed further. 'Meanwhile, literally millions of women suffer the pain and dangers of traditional abortion practices,' he continued, 'yet today, if society wished, it might be on the verge of offering safer and perhaps even self-administered techniques for terminating very early pregnancies.'

Ethically, in whatever way the term is understood, the so-called 'morning after' pill has proved to be much more acceptable, though philosophically one might find little difference between aborting an implanted embryo and aborting an embryo that has merely been just conceived. Estrogens and progestogens are both capable of preventing pregnancy when given shortly after coitus (in medical terms called 'peri-coital' usage), if the dosage is high enough. The hormones act on the uterine lining or tubal motility and thus they upset the sequence of events necessary for implantation, preventing any conception that might have occurred from surviving.

Post-coital pills (in the form of the estrogen ethinyl estradiol 2–5 mg, i.e., several hundred times the normal dosage in one ordinary daily pill, and diethylstilboestrol 25–50 mg, again a massive dose) taken on five consecutive days after unprotected intercourse and beginning within thirty-six hours have achieved a pregnancy rate as low as 0.05%, when otherwise it might have been expected to be as high as 10–20%. Nevertheless, nausea, vomiting and menstrual irregularities ensued, as might be expected from such an overdose of steroid hormones. Another compound with a lower dosage (but perhaps higher potency) is now in favour (namely, levonorgestrel 0.25 mg with 50 microgram of ethinyl estradiol, i.e., not dissimilar to the early 50 microgram combination pill). Two doses are taken: the first within seventy-two hours of the 'risk', and the second twelve hours later. 'If the second dose is forgotten, or lost due to vomiting,' states the UK's Department of Health *Handbook of Contraceptive Practice*, recognising the concomitant side-effects, then 'the complete course should be repeated, if necessary giving anti-emetics. The simplicity of the regimes encourages good compliance. However,' it continues, *'this method is in no sense a substitute for conventional contraceptive practice and is only suitable as an occasional emergency measure.'*

Failure rate is held to be only 1%, but the problem of such an assessment of success is inevitably confused by not knowing if the woman was or was not likely to become pregnant in any case. Isolated acts of unprotected intercourse do not necessarily result in a pregnancy, since it depends so much on the fertility of both partners and the timing of the woman's ovulation. One inherent danger of the 'morning after' dosage is its repetition if the woman decides she does not want to commit herself to the regular use of contraception. So far, the relative safety (or hazards) of repeated use is unknown. Certainly, the dangers of teratological effects (fetal damage) or an ectopic (tubal) pregnancy are recognised. Nevertheless, post-coital pills are marketed widely in Hungary and China (where they are called 'visiting' or 'husband's vacation' pills) and their popularity is growing in the UK.

Quinestrol is an estrogen which is absorbed into body fat and then slowly released over the next three to four weeks. Combined with an oral progesterone it can be used as a once-a-month pill which acts by suppressing ovulation. Its use was pioneered by the Warner-Lambert company in America in the late 1960s but when it was clinically tested in the USA a higher than acceptable pregnancy rate was found, and when further clinical studies showed that a change in the dose of quinestrol was necessary, the potential expense of repeating the whole investment, in trials, research and satisfaction of the drug regulatory authorities, proved too great a deterrent for development to continue. However, in China a formulation of 12 mg of norgestrel with 3 mg of quinestrol has been developed, and its use is recommended as one dose on the fifth day of the woman's menstrual cycle and another on the twelfth. The pregnancy rate appears to be only 2–3% and given that abortion is not only legal but recommended in order to control population growth in the Chinese Peoples' Republic this 'twice a month' pill has proved acceptable. Effects on blood fats, variations in absorption rates depending on body weight, and long-term side-effects are not yet clearly documented but the long-acting steroids such as quinestrol do offer optimistic hope of freedom from the requirement of a daily ritual for contraceptive precautions, to the woman who rates that freedom highly.

OTHER FUTURE DEVELOPMENTS

A new generation of long-acting steroidal contraceptives will enter the market in the 1990s. The FDA in the USA has let it be known that it will accept toxicological and teratological studies which have already been conducted on existing steroids as part of the marketing application for new formulations for steroids. This is more than a mere bureaucratic change and relieves those attempting to introduce new hormonal contraceptives of tens of millions of dollars of research. As a consequence, two non-profit organisations using federal contracts and support from private US foundations are likely to receive marketing approval for subdermal implants and injectables in the early 1990s.

The Population Council in New York has been doing research on Norplants®, which began to be developed in the early 1970s and are silastic rods which release a continuous low dose of levonorgestrel into the bloodstream. Two to six capsules, approximately the size of matchsticks, are inserted under the skin of the upper arm. The device has been demonstrated to give excellent contraceptive protection for five years. It requires a small operation to insert and can be removed at any time if the patient wishes it, or it is taken out at the end of the five years. Removal is sometimes slighly more difficult than insertion.

Biodegradable subdermal implants have also been developed in Family Health International, and the Endocon Corporation are working on a subdermal pellet of norethisterone. The pellet gives one-year protection and can be removed in the first six months of use if the woman is not satisfied, but if it is left in place it biodegrades spontaneously. Family Health International is also working on a three-month injectable using a new, sophisticated formulation which generates tiny spears (about ten times the diameter of a red blood cell) of a mixture of steroid and polylactic acid, the latter being the raw material used in absorbable surgical sutures. By varying the size of the sphere and the mixture of polylactic acid and steroid, various release rates can be obtained, from one month to six months. FDA marketing approval is likely to be given for a three-month injectable in the early 1990s.

All long-acting steroids, with the exception of monthly operations, will cause some disturbance in the menstrual cycle but release directly into the bloodstream is preferable to absorbing the pill through the gut, which overloads the liver with steroid. Exceptionally low blood levels are still associated with contraceptive activity and the absence of estrogen may well reduce or quite possibly totally eliminate the cardio-vascular risks associated with the combined pill.

It is not clear whether these new formulations will be marketed in the USA or whether fear of product liability will prevent them being offered to American women even after they have received FDA approval for marketing. The first product to become available will almost certainly be Norplant®, with the three-monthly injectable a few years behind. The one-year pellets are likely to be the cheapest to produce and may make the greatest impact in the Third World.

Meanwhile, research into other 'non-pill' delivery systems of ovulatory suppressant or fertility control steroids is proceeding perhaps more rapidly. Vaginal rings made of plastic and impregnated with estrogen and progestogen combinations or progestogen alone, and which release a steady dose for absorption, are being developed and assessed. Left in place for up to 3–6 months, or removed whenever conception is planned, they offer a different self-administered method of delivery from the pill. Implants consist of small plastic rods or capsules filled with slow-release hormones, are surgically inserted under the skin and have an effective life of up to five years in maintaining ovulatory suppression. Biodegradable carriers for the hormone are being developed to avoid the necessity for surgical removal of the exhausted implant, but this method nevertheless still suffers the major disadvantage of the requirement for medical intervention in its use. Long-acting injections of the 'depot' hormones are easier to administer, but predictability of the maintenance effect is relatively unreliable.

A 'paper' pill has been developed in China — again where experimentation is so important to achieve cheap, reliable and acceptable preparations. Carboxymethylcellulose paper, which is edible, is dipped into a hormone solution and then dried. Given that the absorbency rate of the paper can be calculated from its area and volume, a sufficient dose is achieved by the consumption of a postage stamp size, perforated from a tear-off strip.

Bearing in mind that most of the standard contraceptive pill consists of an innocuous filler designed to make it big enough to see and handle (and not get lost in the fluff under the bed), the equal dispersion of the small quantities of hormone in each tablet to ensure adequate absorption requires careful quality control. (The Food and Drug Administration of the USA allows an 8% variation in the content, but most manufacturers set higher standards of only 2% variation.)

Packaging in sophisticated 'blister' and calendar labelled packs, marketing, and insurance liability problems render the production costs in the Western world much higher than the actual cost of the constituent hormones themselves. Indeed, the actual cost of hormone production is now less than a tenth of what it was in 1960. In consequence, therefore, it can be seen that the future holds the probability of ever-cheaper forms of delivery of the oral contraceptive hormones being made available to the developing world, and perhaps, ironically, ever-simpler and more convenient packaging of an expensive product in post-coital or monthly pre-menstrual dosage, for the women of the developed world.

Whatever the outcome of current research in the next three decades, unless there is another Russell Marker somewhere in the world currently exploring the capabilities of some hitherto unresearched substance (and it is recognised that there are certain plant extracts from such as *Trichosanthin kirolowii*, yuanhuacine and yuanhuadine, and the Mexican 'tea', *Montana tomentosa* (zoapatle) which have proved abortion-producing activity) no such revolution in the development of oral contraception as that which occurred in 1956 can easily be forecast. The story of the last thirty years has been one of consistent refinement in substance, dosage, delivery and surveillance of effect, a process that is by no means finished yet.

Epilogue

The State of the Art

R. B. Greenblatt

The classic pill enjoyed world-wide acceptance until anecdotal case reports of stroke and pulmonary embolism began to appear[1, 2]. The estrogen component was suspected as being responsible for many trivial reactions, some transient metabolic effects that usually recede when use of the pill is discontinued, and other more serious hazards.

Elimination of the estrogen and use of a progestin only was proposed in 1966 by Martinez–Manautou and co-workers[3]. A large series of cases using 0.5 mg of chlormadinone daily (uninterrupted) showed that this progestin was a moderately effective contraceptive. The failure rate ranged from 3% to 5%. Unfortunately, the development of breast tumours, resembling myoepithelial hyperplasia, in beagles given long-term chlormadinone therapy led the Food and Drug Administration (FDA) to abandon further clinical trials, although no case had been reported following its use in humans. Other progestins, such as norethindrone and norgestrel, did not appear to have tumour-inducing properties in beagles, and miniprogestin pills utilising these two progestins became available for contraception. Aside from a decided reduction in effectiveness, untoward reactions are few; however, a 25% incidence of bleeding irregularities causes many women to discontinue this regimen. Moreover, some proponents of the progestin-only pill have turned full circle and advocated that small doses of estrogens be added to control this undesirable and inconvenient side-effect. A preparation containing 1 mg of norethindrone and 20 μg of ethinyl estradiol* became available but has not

*Trademark: Loestrin® (Parke-Davis, Morris Plains, New Jersey).

been well received because of inadequate performance. It became evident that the classic pill was more dependable and, despite its alleged hazards, the FDA felt that the benefits far outweighed the risks.

THE PILL AND CANCER

Questions were raised that long-term use of the pill might lead to the development of uterine and breast malignancies. Warnings were sounded that the incidence of gynecological cancer would rise precipitously after a latent period of twenty years[4]. The basis for this claim was the finding by Herbst and colleagues[5], in 1971, of vaginal adenosis and occasional clear-cell carcinoma in the daughters of women who had received stilbestrol during pregnancy twenty years earlier. Now that thirty years have elapsed since the introduction of the pill, epidemiological studies reveal that pill-users have, in fact, a lower incidence of endometrial and ovarian cancer. Moreover, no hard facts have appeared to prove an increased incidence of breast tumours[6].

THE PILL AND CARDIO-VASCULAR COMPLICATIONS

Disturbing reports were published by British investigators claiming a close relationship in the rising incidence of a cluster of cardio-vascular complications in pill-users[7]. The reports, reviewed by Mann and Inman[7], suggested links to thrombo-embolism, cerebral thrombosis, and hypertension. Studies[8, 9] by American and other epidemiologists supported the British claims and added myocardial infarction, gallbladder disease, hepatoma, visual defects, and mesenteric thrombosis to the list. Controversy arose as to the interpretation of the collected data, and the subject is still being debated.

Deep vein thrombosis

Case-control and later cohort studies were undertaken to determine the risk factor for deep vein thrombosis. Table 1 (retrospective studies) and Table 2 (prospective studies) list the risk factors for development of deep vein thrombosis in oral contraceptive users[10]. The findings of the different epidemiological studies varied considerably. For instance, in the case-control studies on thrombo-embolism[11] the risk factor varied from 1 to 11, and in cohort studies, from 1.5 to 8.0.

Barnes and colleagues[12] claim that with the use of sophisticated techniques they found that the clinical diagnosis of venous thrombo-embolism was in error in 69% of women not using oral contraceptives, an error that reached 83% in those who did. In our great concern, we failed to consider the natural history of the disease: thrombo-embolism is a much more frequent cause of death than

Table 1 Retrospective studies on deep vein thrombosis in oral contraceptive users★

Investigators	Year	Risk (×)
Royal College of General Practitioners	1967	3.0
Vessey, Doll	1968; 1969	6.3
Inman, Vessey	1968	8.3
Sartwell	1969	4.4
Boston Collaborative Drug Surveillance	1973	11.0
Stolley	1975	7.2

★Data compiled from Guichoux[10]

Table 2 Prospective studies on deep vein thrombosis in oral contraceptive users★

Investigators	Year	Risk (×)
Fuertes de la Habu	1971	1.8
Royal College of General Practitioners	1974	5.6
Kay	1975	5.6
Vessey	1976	2–3
Diddle	1978	1

★Data compiled from Guichoux[10]

hitherto suspected, even in men. Although certain dosages of oral contraceptives do increase the incidence of thrombo-embolism, the weighted incidence is much less than alleged and seems to be negligible in the low-dose pill, as indicated in the Walnut Creek studies undertaken in the USA[13].

Myocardial infarction

Results of the epidemiological studies on thrombo-embolism hold for the other cardio-vascular diseases as well. Following the first publication by Boyce and colleagues[2] in the United Kingdom, concerning myocardial infarction in oral contraceptive users, a rash of individual case reports appeared in many other scientific journals throughout the world. It was only after publication of the Oxford Family Planning study[14, 15] that the problem began to be considered seriously outside the United Kingdom. These findings received ready corroboration in the United States. Jain[16], however, refuted the British studies and injected the concept that there was a strong association between cigarette smoking and mortality in oral contraceptive users (Table 3). Others suggested, as Jain had done, that myocardial infarction was caused more by smoking than by the pill.

Table 3 Mortality associated with pregnancy and childbirth, legal abortion, and oral contraceptives in smokers and non-smokers in women of different ages

Age range (years)	Pregnancy and childbirth*	Legal abortion†	Oral contraceptives‡	
			Non-smokers	Smokers
15–19	11.1	1.2	1.2	1.4
20–24	10.0	1.2	1.2	1.4
25–29	12.5	1.4	1.2	1.4
30–34	24.9	1.4	1.8	10.4
35–39	44.0	1.8	3.9	12.8
40–44	71.4	1.8	6.6	58.4

* Per 100 000 live births (excluding abortion), USA, 1972–1974
† Per 100 000 first trimester abortions, USA, 1972–1974
‡ Per 100 000 users/year. Estimates by Dr Anrudh K. Jain[16]

The studies of the Oxford Group[14, 15] also suggested an increased risk of myocardial mortality and morbidity in pill-users, especially in women over the age of 35. In analysing the clinical history of the nine women who died of cardio-vascular disease, as reported by Vessey and colleagues[14] in 1977, it appears that three had previous heart disease, three had a history of toxemia, seven of the nine were smokers, and all but two were aged 35 or more. Although certainly not a momentous series, it put fear in the hearts of physicians who did not study the data (Table 4). In their continued cohort studies[15], seven more deaths were recorded: four myocardial deaths in occasional pill users, all smokers, occurred 18, 50, 84 and 96 months after cessation of pill use in women aged 44, 32, 46, and 44 years, respectively. Each woman had a poor medical history: one had hypertension and had undergone bypass surgery; another had pre-eclampsia with inhalation of vomit; one had hypertension; and another had toxemia.

Table 4 Clinical histories of nine oral contraceptive users who died of cardio-vascular disease[13]

Clinical history	No. of patients	Cigarettes smoked/day	Ages (years)
Heart disease Mitral valve disease Bundle branch block at age 27 Fallot's tetralogy	3	12, 0, 5	43, 37, 32
Toxemia	3	20, 20, 20	37, 36, 28
None	3	17, 15, 0	37, 36, 35

More recent reports by the two major groups in the United Kingdom are far less alarming, and it appears that the investigators are having second thoughts. At one time, a limitation on the length of contraceptive use was suggested. The latest Royal College of General Practitioners study[17] admits, 'We no longer find an increasing risk of death due to vascular disease with increasing duration of the pill.' Furthermore, Vessey and colleagues[15] of the Oxford group commented, 'Our findings do not suggest that the pill is a cause of subarachnoid hemorrhage.'

Certain epidemiological studies, well intentioned as they may be, have created an atmosphere of fear and anxiety. This climate is not easily dislodged, despite the assurances given by such distinguished epidemiologists as the late Dr Tietze[18], who repeatedly pointed out the many erroneous conclusions of certain surveys. Wiseman and MacRae[19] analysed the complexity of the problem and concluded that the risk estimates of serious cardio-vascular problems derived from reports in the United States and in Great Britain are gross overestimates, echoing the beliefs recently expressed by Speroff[20] regarding American studies.

EVOLUTION OF LOW-DOSAGE ORAL CONTRACEPTIVES

The first generation of the classic or combined pill contained considerably more estrogen and progestin than was necessary for conception control. Reports from the United Kingdom implicated the estrogen component in the development of such adverse reactions as hypertension, myocardial infarction, and stroke. Lower estrogen doses were advocated, resulting in preparations containing only 50 μg of ethinyl estradiol in the belief that such a dosage would lessen the risks of cardio-vascular and cerebro-vascular accidents[21, 22]. Inman and colleagues[23] showed a dose–response relationship between estrogen doses > 50 μg and death from thrombo-embolism. They believed that oral contraceptives containing ≤ 50 μg of estrogen might reduce the risk appreciably. According to Mishell and associates[24], thrombo-embolic mortality is at least halved when the amount of synthetic estrogen is reduced from 100 to 50 μg.

Meade and colleagues[25], in 1980, claimed a lower incidence of ischemic heart disease and death when a 30-μg dose of the estrogen was used, and related the incidence of stroke to the high progestin count. As a consequence, a new series of combination pills containing 30 to 35 μg of ethinyl estradiol and low doses of progestin was

130

introduced. These proved as effective as those containing 50 μg in preventing pregnancy.

Reductions in dosage followed the accepted principle to use as little of a therapeutic agent as possible to achieve desired results. Though Edelman and his colleagues[21] found that women using low-dosage oral contraceptives experienced fewer side-effects (nausea, vomiting, headaches, breast tenderness), the increased frequency of break-through bleeding adversely affected continuation rates. For this reason, the 30 and 35 μg pills have not completely replaced the 50 μg compounds (Table 5).

In an effort to lessen untoward reactions, Lachnit-Fixson[26], at Schering in West Germany, devised a preparation in the early 1970s employing a biphasic concept adapted to the phases of the menstrual cycle (Figure 1A). In the United States, Ortho Pharmaceuticals intro-

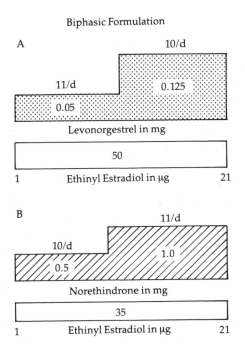

Figure 1 Biphasic oral contraceptives

Table 5 Estrogen and progestin contents of low–dose and very–low–dose oral contraceptives

Drug*	Estrogen	μg	Progestin
A. Low-dose oral contraceptives			
Demulen® (Searle)	Ethinyl estradiol	50	Ethynodiol acetate
Ovral® (Wyeth)	Ethinyl estradiol	50	Norgestrel
Norlestrin® 2.5/50 (Parke–Davis)	Ethinyl estradiol	50	Norethindrone acetate
Norlestrin® 1/50 (Parke–Davis)	Ethinyl estradiol	50	Norethindrone acetate
Ovcon®-50 (Mead Johnson)	Ethinyl estradiol	50	Norethindrone
Noriny1® 1 + 50 (Syntex)	Mestranol	50	Norethindrone
Ortho–Novum® 1/50 (Ortho)	Mestranol	50	Norethindrone
B. Very-low-dose oral contraceptives			
Demulen® 1/35 (Searle)	Ethinyl estradiol	35	Ethynodiol diacetate
Noriny1® + 35 (Syntex)	Ethinyl estradiol	35	Norethindrone
Ortho–Novum® 1/35 (Ortho)	Ethinyl estradiol	35	Norethindrone
Brevicon® (Syntex)	Ethinyl estradiol	35	Norethindrone
Modicon® (Ortho)	Ethinyl estradiol	35	Norethindrone
Ovcon®-35 (Mead Johnson)	Ethinyl estradiol	35	Norethindrone
Lo/Ovral® (Wyeth)	Ethinyl estradiol	30	Norgestrel
Loestrin® 1.5/30 (Parke–Davis)	Ethinyl estradiol	30	Norethindrone acetate
Nordette® (Wyeth)	Ethinyl estradiol	30	Levonorgestrel

* US approved trade names

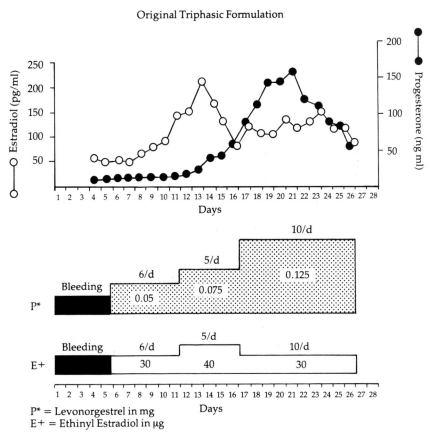

Figure 2 The triphasic oral contraceptive. (Adapted from Lachnit-Fixson[26])

duced the biphasic concept of 35 μg of ethinyl estradiol and 0.5 mg of norethindrone for the first 10 days with an increase to 1 mg of norethindrone for the last 11 days of the 21-day course (Figure 1B).

A further step, imaginative and innovative, in which the triphasic formulation imitated even more closely the fluctuations of estrogen and progesterone of the normal cycle (Figure 2) was introduced in Europe in 1979[26]. The first phase consisted of six days of 30 μg of ethinyl estradiol and 0.05 mg of levonorgestrel; the second phase consisted of five days of 40 μg of ethinyl estradiol and 0.075 mg of levonorgestrel; and the third phase consisted of 30 μg of ethinyl estradiol and 0.125 mg of levonorgestrel. The increased ethinyl estradiol in the second phase was meant to harmonise with the preovulatory surge of E_2 in the normal ovulatory cycle, and the increased levonorgestrel in the third phase was in accord with the luteal levels of progesterone. The rationale for this 'hormone balancing' appears logical and is a further attempt at a more physiological approach. Three triphasic formulations are now available in the United States (Table 6).

Inhibition of ovulation and pregnancy rates

Both estrogens and progestins in adequate dosage inhibit ovulation in a high percentage of trials; each by itself is not a completely reliable suppressor of ovulation. This is one of the reasons why pregnancy rates were slightly higher following use of the original sequential than with the combination pill. Because there is a synergistic action between progestin and estrogen, low dosages of both components

Table 6 Triphasic oral contraceptives available in the United States

Drug	Estrogen	μg	Progestin	μg
Triphasil®*/Trinordiol®†				
6 days	Ethinyl estradiol	30	Levonorgestrel	0.050
5 days	Ethinyl estradiol	40	Levonorgestrel	0.075
10 days	Ethinyl estradiol	30	Levonorgestrel	0.125
Ortho-Novum® 7/7/7 (Ortho)				
10 days	Ethinyl estradiol	35	Norethindrone	0.50
7 days	Ethinyl estradiol	35	Norethindrone	0.75
7 days	Ethinyl estradiol	35	Norethindrone	1.00
Tri-Norinyl® (Syntex)				
7 days	Ethinyl estradiol	35	Norethindrone	0.50
9 days	Ethinyl estradiol	35	Norethindrone	1.00
5 days	Ethinyl estradiol	35	Norethindrone	0.50

* US trademark
† European trademark

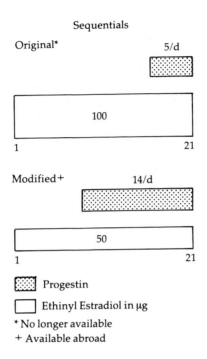

Sequentials

Original*   5/d

100

1   21

Modified+   14/d

50

1   21

Progestin

Ethinyl Estradiol in µg

* No longer available
+ Available abroad

Figure 3   Sequential oral contraceptives

successfully inhibit ovulation; as little as 30–35 µg of ethinyl estradiol may be used with a progestin. Furthermore, the progestin acts as a back-up by increasing the viscosity of the cervical mucus, thus creating a barrier to sperm penetration.

It is now appreciated that the original sequential pill contained too high an estrogen dose (100 µg of ethinyl estradiol or 80 µg of mestranol) and too short a course of progestin. Modified sequentials, in which a dose of 50 µg of ethinyl estradiol is given for seven days followed by a combination of the estrogen and a progestin for 14 or 15 days, may find a place in contraception because this formulation also imitates the hormonal changes of the normal cycle (Figure 3).

Theoretically, the triphasic pill should be as effective a contraceptive as the low-dose uniphasic, the biphasic, or the modified sequential compounds; available statistics substantiate that it is. In a collective experience, based on the use of Triphasil® in 50 000 cycles, Upton[27] reports eight pregnancies (only one of which was a method failure).

Equally good results have been claimed for the other triphasic pills. Pasquale[28], reporting on the collective data obtained from investigators in the United States, Canada, and France with Ortho-Novum® 7/7/7, showed that patients using this preparation had less breakthrough bleeding than did patients on biphasic therapy and that the bleeding pattern was similar to that observed for Ortho-Novum® 1/35. Side-effects were infrequent, and the metabolic impact was low. The incidence of on-pill amenorrhea was 1.2%. The contraceptive efficiency was equal to that of the higher dose contraceptives[28]. Similar reports have surfaced concerning the use of Tri-Norinyl®. Edgren[29], quoting Bradley and colleagues on the Walnut Creek data[30], speculated that norethindrone-based triphasics have a slightly more favourable impact on lipid metabolism than do those containing levonorgestrel.

Cycle control and intermenstrual or midcycle breakthrough bleeding

A formulation that takes into consideration the rapid ovulatory estrogen surge and the slower and sustained postovulatory rise in progesterone secretion of the normal ovulatory cycle theoretically should avoid midcycle and intermenstrual bleeding. Certainly the increasing dosage of the progestin in three stages is based on good physiological principles. A parallel may be found when menses is held in abeyance after conception because of the rising levels of progesterone in the presence of adequate estrogens.

As long ago as 1959, I[31] demonstrated the concept of increasing doses of a progestin to prevent progesterone breakthrough bleeding. In amenorrheic women with adequate endogenous estrogens, a five-day course of 1 mg of norethindrone induces a withdrawal period 24 to 72 hours after the last dose. In a small number of women, breakthrough bleeding occurs by the fourth day of treatment. This can be avoided by increasing the progestin dose. If the new dosage is extended for ten days, withdrawal bleeding occurs 24 to 72 hours later, but breakthrough bleeding occurs in a few by the eighth or ninth day of treatment. If the dosage is again increased, no breakthrough bleeding occurs and the drug may be continued for weeks or months. Two of the three triphasic contraceptive pills currently available in the United States (Triphasil and Ortho-Novum 7/7/7) follow the principle of increasing the dosage of progestin in three stages, whereas Tri-Norinyl has a midcycle increase of progestin for nine days, then decreases for the last five days. This formulation is conceptually different from the other two triphasics. However, the rate of break-through bleeding is relatively low with each of the three triphasic preparations. Statistics show that after the third cycle breakthrough bleeding rarely occurs.

Progestin potency

Much has been written in recent years about potency of progesterone-like drugs. While it is true that the total progestin dosage in Triphasil/Trinordiol is lower than that in other triphasics, consideration should be given to the fact that levonorgestrel, milligram for milligram, is far more potent than norethindrone. It is difficult to compare potencies of progestins because there are decidedly different endpoints. For instance, the amount of a progestin needed to delay the onset of menses[32] is far different when 50 to 100 μg of ethinyl estradiol is added to the progestin[33]. Whether the Greenblatt test[32] or the Swyer modification[33] is a better index of potency is debatable. At best, the tests are imprecise and afford only some idea of relative potency if the particular criterion is the delay of menses[34]. If the arrest of dysfunctional bleeding is used as an index of progestinal potency, norethindrone is more than twice as effective as medroxyprogesterone, milligram for milligram, but far less than norgestrel.

In the study of pharmacological agents there are different parameters to be considered. For instance, in the evaluation of such corticoids as dexamethasone, hydrocortisone, and fludrocortisone, the first is by far the most potent gluco-corticoid, the last the most potent salt

Table 7 Clinical histories of patients with post-pill or on-pill related amenorrhea-galactorrhea*

Patient	Age (years)	Parity	Age at menarche (years)	Previous cycle (days)	Oral Contraceptive	Duration (months)		
						Therapy	Amenorrhea	Galactorrhea
Post-pill								
GC	24	1	13	28–42	Norethindrone, 2 mg, Mestranol, 100 µg	31	14	21†
VG	26	0	11	28	Norethindrone, 2 mg, Mestranol, 100 µg	15	48	52†
DS	23	0	13	Irregular	Norethindrone, 2 mg, Mestranol, 100 µg	12	7	7
LT	26	1	11	28	?	36	48	48
CS	29	1	12	30	Combined	8	51	‡
On-pill								
GP	34	Abl	11	Amenorrhea§	Norethynodrel, 2.5 mg, Mestranol, 100 µg	42	72	72
PW	29	0	12	Amenorrhea§	?	30	30	‡
DM	27	0	12	Amenorrhea§	Chlormadinone, 2 mg, Mestranol, 80 µg	48	48	60†
SH	32	1	14	Amenorrhea§	Norethynodrel, 5 mg, Mestranol, 75 µg	6	54	‡
LB	26	0	14½	Amenorrhea§	Chlormadinone, 2 mg, Mestranol, 80 µg	24	36	‡

* Adapted from Gambrell and colleagues[38]
† Galactorrhea onset while taking pills
‡ Galactorrhea detected on initial physical examination
§ Had fairly regular cycles before onset of amenorrhea

retainer, a property that is important in the management of Addison's disease. Thus, too, in the original delay of menses test (without the addition of an estrogen) 0.5 mg of norgestrel and 15 mg of norethindrone administered from day 20 to day 40 could, in the majority of trials, delay the onset of menses to the 42nd day. The larger doses of norethindrone need not necessarily imply that the risks are greater or that the lower doses of levonorgestrel are less.

In the last analysis, the delay of menses tests, glycogen deposition, ovulation inhibition, induction of withdrawal bleeding, and depression of the vaginal karyopyknotic index are not conclusive standards of reference. Each of these tests is a comparative rather than an absolute expression of drug activity. What is of greater importance is that the low-dose estrogen/progestin formulation be effective in contraceptive and cycle control with minimal lipid and other metabolic changes[35].

Pill-related galactorrhea and amenorrhea

One of the undesirable effects of oral contraceptives is the occurrence of pill-related amenorrhea, which often is accompanied by galactorrhea. Failure to respond with a menstrual flow after termination of pill use is observed more frequently in women who had irregular menses before taking the pill. Such happenings are believed to result from temporary derangement of hypothalamic-pituitary function, which usually corrects itself within six months[36]. The amenorrhea, however, may last for years and compromise chances for fertility[37]. We[38] have encountered patients in whom the amenorrhea had already been present for seven to 72 months, especially when associated with galactorrhea (Table 7)[37]. Whether the amenorrhea and galactorrhea syndrome is due to an unsuspected prolactinoma that becomes manifest after termination of pill use or merely represents induced pituitary dysfunction is debatable. March and colleagues[39] do not consider oral contraceptives responsible.

I have been interested in inappropriate galactorrhea for some 40 years and encountered relatively few cases before the advent of oral contraceptives. Then, within a decade or two, reports of this unusual finding inundated the literature. Since the dosage of the pill has been greatly reduced there appears to be a corresponding decline in the incidence of galactorrhea, amenorrhea, and on-pill amenorrhea. There may be a good physiological reason for such a sequence of events. The low-dose pill is gentler on pituitary suppression. Based on the work of Spellacy and colleagues[40], Upton[41] speculated that the triphasic pill with its low steroid content would not cause as much pituitary suppression as would the classic pill. De Cecco and his colleagues[42] have demonstrated that the supposition was bona fide. Return of pituitary responsiveness to a gonadotropin-releasing hormone challenge test was more rapid after the triphasic pill than after the regular uniphasic pill (Figure 4). Of 22 768 cycles studied in

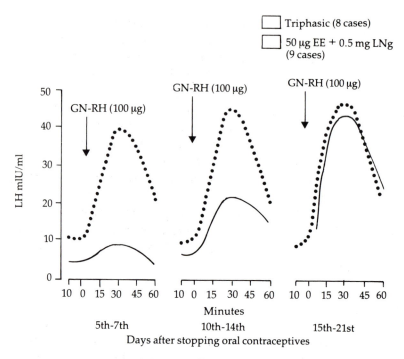

Figure 4 Pituitary response to gonadotropin-releasing hormone (GnRH) after stopping contraceptive pills. (Adapted from De Cecco and colleagues[42])

women on one of the triphasic pills, fewer than 0.3% failed to have withdrawal bleeding[27].

Many investigators have shown that oral contraceptives are capable of preventing the surge of luteinising hormone while causing a rise in prolactin secretion, due perhaps to suppression of prolactin-inhibiting factor. The estrogen-dominant pill usually induces greater prolactin release than does the progestin-dominant pill[43]. Nonetheless, the effect varies among individuals receiving the same oral contraceptive. According to Mishell and colleagues[44], this idiosyncrasy may be related to the development of the syndrome of galactorrhea. In a follow-up study he and his associates[45] found that the basal and the maximal prolactin response to protirelin was greater in subjects using oral contraceptives than in controls; however, they reported no difference in prolactin response in subjects on the high or low estrogen dosage pill.

Although the administration of natural estrogens in physiological doses does not appear to increase serum prolactin levels, large doses do[46]. We noted that the original oral contraceptives raised prolactin to higher levels than those following large doses of estradiol 17-beta in the form of pellet implantation (Figure 5).

The question of the relationship between oral contraceptives and galactorrhea and amenorrhea remains a perplexing one. The Mayo Clinic group[47] found a direct link between pill discontinuation and galactorrhea but none attributable to pill use itself. They feel the mechanism for this is unknown. In comparison with a reference group who had never used the pill, women who had ever used the pill were found to be two to three times more likely to have galactorrhea. The investigators believe that bias may have been introduced into their study because women using the pill tend to be seen more often by physicians than do non-users.

QUESTION OF LIPIDS

Lipoproteins are affected differently by estrogens and progestins: estrogens increase high density lipoproteins (HDL), and progestins increase low density lipoproteins (LDL). Relatively high levels of

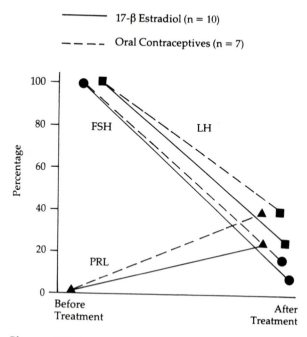

——————— 17-β Estradiol (n = 10)

– – – – Oral Contraceptives (n = 7)

Figure 5 Changes (%) in serum concentrations of follicle-stimulating hormone (FSH), luteinising hormone (LH), and prolactin (PRL) after six months of oral contraceptive use as compared with that of implanted estradiol pellets. The oral contraceptive pill induced slightly higher prolactin levels than that following estradiol pellets used in a sequential type of contraception

LDL-cholesterol are associated with a high incidence of coronary artery disease, while high levels of HDL-cholesterol, it is claimed, are protective. The early progestin-dominant oral contraceptives have been incriminated; some progestins decrease HDL or increase LDL more so than others[48]. A comparison of the oral contraceptive users versus non-users in the Framingham study[49] indicated that total plasma cholesterol, triglycerides, and very low density lipoproteins (VLDL) were significantly elevated in pill-users, while HDL and LDL were not significantly changed. Early case-control studies conducted by the Boston Collaborative Drug Surveillance Program[50] in the early 1970s revealed a high risk of venous thrombo–embolism, myocardial infarction, and stroke. Age, smoking, and predisposing illness contributed to the risk factors. Recent studies[50] indicate that women using the low-dose oral contraceptives are at very low risk, if any, for stroke or myocardial infarction. In studies of women on the ethinyl estradiol/ levonorgestrel triphasic, no significant change was seen in lipid parameters at eighteen months. The HDL-cholesterol ratios to total cholesterol and to LDL-cholesterol were not statistically different from baseline values. In a study by Rabe and colleagues[51] of the triphasic pill containing norethindrone, little change was found in lipid patterns, including apolipoproteins AI, AII and B. Notelovitz and colleagues[52], using conventional low-dose oral contraceptives such as one containing 0.4 mg of norethindrone and 35 μg of ethinyl estradiol, found serum cholesterol, HDL-cholesterol, LDL-cholesterol, and triglyceride levels unchanged. In our experience[53], we found that if a potent estrogen in used, HDL is slightly increased and LDL and VLDL are slightly decreased regardless of the progestin used (Figure 6).

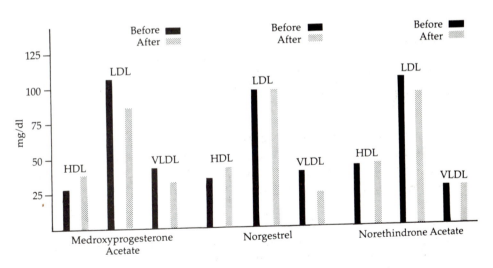

Figure 6 Comparison of serum lipoproteins six months after implantation of 100 mg of estradiol pellets. Progestins given for ten days each month to induce orderly withdrawal periods were medroxyprogesterone acetate (10 mg) in 29, norgestrel (0.075 mg) in 15, and norethindrone acetate (5 mg) in 10 patients. HDL levels were slightly increased with little change in VLDL and LDL values

CONCLUSION

Ever since humans became aware of the relationship between coitus and conception, they have searched for some method — mechanical, medicinal, or magical — to prevent pregnancy or limit the number of progeny. Conception control has served to unfetter women from the fears of an unwanted pregnancy and thus has done much to improve the morale and well-being of the women who practise it. Limitation of family size to the desired number of children is good both for the family unit and for society. Every child should be wanted and planned for, with a design for his or her future welfare.

Closely allied to this theme of birth control is the greater and weightier problem of national and international concern — the population explosion. High-density populations foster social stress, poverty, hostility, violence and moral degradation.

For several years there has been a trend away from the pill because of the increased mortality rates, particularly in pill-users over 35 years of age and in those who smoke. Epidemiological studies have shown that the incidence of death from cardio-vascular disease, thrombo-embolic disease, and stroke was reduced greatly as the steroidal content of the pill was reduced. The reduction of the estrogen component from 150 μg of ethinyl estradiol-3-methylether (mestranol) to 30–35 μg of ethinyl estradiol and of the progestin component from 10 mg of norethindrone to 1 mg or less has not interfered with effective conception control nor to any extent with cycle control, yet it has minimised untoward effects. It is now more apparent that the progestin component of the pill was linked to high blood pressure, lipid changes, and cardio-vascular disturbances with an unfavourable impact on arterial disease. According to an editorial by Roland and Edgren[54], the question whether oral contraceptives cause or pre-dispose to cardio-vascular problems cannot be answered at this time. They feel that the risks attributable to these drugs are very small indeed and are markedly outweighed by the benefits.

With new formulations that more closely imitate the hormonal fluctuations of the menstrual cycle, the progestin contents of both norethindrone and levonorgestrel are at a level that augurs nothing but good for the pill-user. Triphasic formulations hold much promise as to safety and effectiveness. Whether these offer advantages over the low-dose oral contraceptives remains to be determined. Progestins are now viewed as the bête noire of the oral contraceptives. Certainly one point cannot be disputed: the total progestin in the triphasic pill is lower than in the low-dose uniphasic or biphasic pill. Perhaps Kay's[55] characterisation of the new low-dose pill as the 'happiness pill' will prove prophetic.

This chapter is from an article by R. B. Greenblatt which was first published in *Current Therapeutics*.

REFERENCES

1. Jordan, W. M. (1962). Pulmonary embolism. *Lancet*, **2**, 1146
2. Boyce, J., Fawcett, J. W. and Noall, E. W. O. (1963). Coronary thrombosis and conovid. *Lancet*, **2**, 111
3. Martinez-Manautou, J., Ramos, R. A. and Giner, J. (1974). The premenopausal woman: Her fear of pregnancy and choice of contraceptives. In Greenblatt, R. B., Mahesh, V. B. and McDonough, P. G. (eds) *The Menopausal Syndrome*, p. 162. Medcom Press, New York
4. Hertz, R. in discussion of Greenblatt, R. B. (1972). Nuovi sviluppi della contraccezione steroidea. In Pascetto, G. and De Cecco, L. (eds) *Controllo della Fecondita*, p. 309. Edizione Minerva Medici, Genoa
5. Herbst, A. L., Ulfelder, H. and Poskanzer, D. C. (1971). Adenocarcinoma of the vagina. Association of maternal stilbestrol therapy with tumor appearance in young women. *N. Engl. J. Med.*, **284**, 878
6. Ory, H. W. (1983). Oral contraceptive use and risk of breast cancer. Oral contraceptive use and risk of ovarian cancer. The Centers for Disease Control Cancer and Steroid Hormone Study. *J. Am. Med. Assoc.*, **249**, 1591–600
7. Marin, J. I. and Inman, W. H. W. (1975). Oral contraceptives and death from myocardial infarction. *Br. Med. J.*, **2**, 245
8. Rosenberg, L. (1976). Myocardial infarction and estrogen therapy

in premenopausal women. *N. Engl. J. Med.*, **294**, 1290

9. Jick, H. *et al.* (1978). Oral contraceptives and nonfatal myocardial infarction. *J. Am. Med. Assoc.*, **238**, 1403

10. Guichoux, J. Y. (ed.) (1979). *Bilan Medical des Traitments Oestro-progestatifs.* Maloine SA Editeur, Paris

11. Vessey, M. P. *et al.* (1980). Female hormones and vascular disease: An epidemiological review. *Br. J. Fam. Plan.*, **6**, (Suppl. 1), 1–12

12. Barnes, R. W., Krapt, T. and Hoak, J. C. (1978). Erroneous clinical diagnosis of leg and vein thrombosis in women on oral contraceptives. *Obstet. Gynecol.*, **51**, 556

13. Ramcharan, S., Pellegrin, F. A., Ray, R. M. *et al.* (1980). The Walnut Creek Contraceptive Drug Study: A prospective study of the side effects of oral contraceptives: A comparison of disease occurrence leading to hospitalization or death in users and non-users of oral contraceptives. *J. Reprod. Med.*, **25**, (Suppl.), 345

14. Vessey, M. P., McPherson, K. and Johnson, B. (1977). Mortality among women participating in the Oxford Family Planning Association contraceptive study. *Lancet*, **2**, 731

15. Vessey, M. P., McPherson, K. and Yeates, D. (1981). Mortality in oral contraceptive users. *Lancet*, **1**, 549

16. Jain, A. K. (1976). Cigarette smoking, use of oral contraceptives, and myocardial infarction. *Am. J. Obstet. Gynecol.*, **136**, 301

17. Royal College of General Practitioners (1977). Effect of hypertension and benign breast disease of progestogen component in combined oral contraceptives. *Lancet*, **2**, 624

18. Tietze, C. (1979). The pill and mortality from cardiovascular disease: Another look. *Fam. Plan. Perspect.*, **11**, 80

19. Wiseman, R. A. and MacRae, K. D. (1981). Oral contraceptives and the decline in mortality from circulatory disease. *Fertil. Steril.*, **35**, 277

20. Speroff, L. (1982). The formulation of oral contraceptives: Does the amount of estrogen make any clinical difference? *Johns Hopkins Med. J.*, **150**, 170–6

21. Edelman, D. A., Kothenbeutel, R., Levinski, M. J. *et al.* (1983). Comparative trials of low-dose combined oral contraceptives. *J. Reprod. Med.*, **28**, 195

22. Inman, W. H. and Vessey, M. P. (1968). Investigation of deaths from pulmonary, coronary, and cerebral thrombosis and embolism in women of child-bearing age. *Br. Med. J.*, **2**, 193

23. Inman, W. H., Vessey, M. P., Westerholm, B. *et al.* (1970). Thromboembolic disease and the steroidal content of oral contraceptives. A report of the Committee of Safety of Drugs. *Br. Med. J.*, **2**, 203

24. Mishell, D. R., Brenner, P. F., Chez, R. A. *et al.* (1982). Oral contraception today. Three dialogues. *J. Reprod. Med.*, **27**, (Suppl. 4), 235

25. Meade, T. W., Greenburg, G. and Thompson, S. G. (1980). Progestogens and cardiovascular reactions associated with oral contraceptives and a comparison of the safety of 50- and 35-μg oestrogen preparations. *Br. Med. J.*, **280**, 1157

26. Lachnit-Faxson, U. (1980). The rationale for a new triphasic contraceptive. In Greenblatt, R. B. (ed.) *The Development of a New Triphasic Oral Contraceptive*, p. 23. MTP Press Ltd, Lancaster

27. Upton, V. (1983). The phasic approach to oral contraception. *Int. J. Fertil.*, **28**, 121

28. Pasquale, S. A. (1984). Rationale for a triphasic oral contraceptive. *J. Reprod. Med.*, **29**, (Suppl.), 560

29. Edgren, R. A. (1985). Introduction. In *Lipoproteins, Exogenous Steroids, and Cardiovascular Problems*, pp 4–5. Syntex Laboratories, Inc., Palo Alto, California

30. Bradley, D. D., Wingerd, J., Petitti, D. B. *et al.* (1978). Serum high density-lipoprotein cholesterol in women using oral contraceptives, estrogens and progestins. *N. Engl. J. Med.*, **299**, 17–20

31. Greenblatt, R. B. (1959). Hormonal control of functional uterine bleeding. *Clin. Obstet. Gynecol.*, **2**, 232

32. Greenblatt, R. B., Clark, S. L. and Jungek, E. C. (1958). A new test for efficacy of progestational agents. *Ann. NY Acad. Sci.*, **71**, 717

33. Swyer, G. I. M. (1982). Potency of progestogens in oral contraceptives — further delay of menses data. *Contraception*, **26**, 23

34. Gilmer, M. D. G. (1984). The relevance of potency tests. *J. Obstet. Gynecol.*, **4**, (Suppl. 2), 128

35. Newton, J. (1984). Pills in perspective: Practical aspects of pre-scribing. *J. Obstet. Gynecol.*, **4**, (Suppl. 2), 139
36. Pettersson, F., Fries, H. and Nillius, S. J. (1973). Epidemiology of secondary amenorrhea. 1. Incidence and prevalent rate. *Am. J. Obstet. Gynecol.*, **117**, 80
37. Vessey, M. P., Doll, R., Peto, R. *et al.* (1976). A long-term follow-up study of women using different methods of contra-ception. An interim report. *J. Biosocial Sci.*, **8**, 373
38. Gambrell, R. D., Greenblatt, R. B. and Mahesh, V. (1971). Post-pill and pill related amenorrhea-galactorrhea. *Am. J. Obstet. Gynecol.*, **110**, 838
39. March, C. M., Mishell, D. R., Jr. and Kletzky, O. A. (1979). Galactorrhea and pituitary tumors in postpill and non-postpill secondary amenorrhea. *Am. J. Obstet. Gynecol.*, **134** (1), 45–8
40. Spellacy, W. H., Kalra, P. S., Buhi, W. C. and Birk, S. A. (1980). Pituitary and ovarian responsiveness to a graded gonadotropin releasing factor stimulation-test in women using a low-estrogen type of oral contraceptive. *Am. J. Obstet. Gynecol.*, **137**, 109
41. Upton, G. V. (1980). The normal menstrual cycle and oral contraceptives: The physiologic basis for a triphasic approach. In Greenblatt, R. B. (ed.) *The Development of the New Triphasic Oral Contraceptive*, pp 11–49. MTP Press Ltd, Lancaster
42. De Cecco, L., Capitanio, G., Venturini, P. *et al.* (1982). The effi-cacy of triphasic oral contraceptives and effects on the pituitary-ovarian axis in younger women compared with older types of contraceptives. In Brosens, J. (ed.) *New Considerations in Oral Contraception*, pp 191–208. Biomedical Information Corp., New York
43. Abu-Fadil, S., Devane, G., Siber, T. M. and Yen, S. S. C. (1976). Effects of oral contraceptive steroids on pituitary prolactin secretion. *Contraception*, **13**, 79
44. Mishell, D. R., Jr., Kletzky, D. H., Brenner, P. F. *et al.* (1977). The effect of contraceptive steroids on hypothalamic pituitary function. *Am. J. Obstet. Gynecol.*, **128**, 60
45. Scott, J. Z., Kletzky, D. A., Brenner, P. F. and Mishell, D. R., Jr. (1978). Comparison of the effects of contraceptive steroid formu-

lations containing two doses of estrogen on pituitary function. *Fertil. Steril.*, **30**, 141

46. Ben David, M. and L'Hermite, M. (1973). Prolactin and menopause. In van Keep, P. A., Greenblatt, R. B. and Albeaux-Fernet (eds) *Consensus on Menopause Research*, p. 48. MTP Press Ltd, Lancaster

47. Coulam, C. B., Thaler, S. J., Annegers, J. F. and Brittain, E. (1984). Case-control study of galactorrhea and its relationship to the use of oral contraceptives. Presented at the annual meeting of the American Fertility Society, 4–9 April, New Orleans

48. (1985). *Lipoproteins, Exogenous Steroids, and Cardiovascular Problems*. Syntex Laboratories, Inc., Palo Alto, California

49. Castelli, W. P. (1985). Effects of exogenous steroids: The Framingham experience. In *Lipoproteins, Exogenous Steroids, and Cardiovascular Problems*, p. 53. Syntex Laboratories, Inc., Palo Alto, California

50. Jick, H. (1985). Epidemiology of oral contraceptive-related cardiovascular disease. In *Lipoproteins, Exogenous Steroids, and Cardiovascular Problems*, p. 61. Syntex Laboratories, Inc., Palo Alto, California

51. Rabe, T., Runebaum, B., Hageloch, X. *et al.* (1984). Influence of norethindrone containing triphasic pill on carbohydrate and lipids. *Metab. Contracept. Delivery Syst.*, **5** 50

52. Notelovitz, M., Gudal, J. and McKenzie, I. C. (1981). *Contraceptives, lipids, and lipoproteins. The metabolic effects of a low estrogen, low progestin oral contraceptive*, p. 20. Biomedical Information Corp., New York

53. Greenblatt, R. B., Chadda, J. S., Teran, A. Z. and Nezhat, C. (1984). Estrogens: Whence, when, why, how. *Today's Ther. Trends*, **2**, 27

54. Roland, M. and Edgren, R. A. (1984). Editorial. *Int. J. Fertil.*, **29**

55. Kay, C. R. (1980). The happiness pill? *J. Roy. Coll. Gen. Pract.*, **30**, 8

Index

abortion, 15, 41, 99
abortion-producing agents, 119–21, 124
amenorrhea, pill-related, 139–41

beagle dog, tests on, 73–4, 90, 125
biphasic pills, 131, 133, 145
breakthrough bleeding, 36, 131, 136–7
breastfeeding, effects of, 13, 20, 88–9,
    100, 102

cancer
    breast, 73–4, 100, 101–3, 125
    correlation with childbearing and
        ovulation, 100–2
    fears of, 52, 97–8
    risk of, 86, 90, 97, 126
        breast, 56, 91, 100–3, 126
        endometrial, 57, 93, 94, 97, 100,
          101, 102, 126
        ovarian, 57, 93, 94, 97, 100, 101,
          102, 126
        uterine cervix, 56, 94
cardio-vascular disease, 53, 56, 57, 71–2,
    90, 93, 94, 97, 99–100, 123,
    126–30, 142–3, 144
Chang, M.C., 33–4, 87
chemical formulae of ovarian hormones,
    26
Colton, Frank D., 33
contraception
    change in attitude of medical
        profession towards, 39–41, 43
    early methods of, 13–20
    legality of, 20–1, 34

contraceptive methods
    availability of, 86
    general perceptions of, 46–50
corpus luteum, 23, 78–9
cortisone, synthesis of, 25, 27, 30
cyproterone-acetate, 117

death
    due to fertility regulation, 99–100
    due to pill usage, 37, 90, 99–100,
        106–8, 129
    due to pregnancy, 94–6, 99–100, 103
Depo-Provera, 90, 92, 102
diosgenin, 27, 28, 30
Djerassi, Carl, 29–31

epidemiological studies, 55, 56, 67, 91,
    100–3, 126–30
estradiol
    chemical formula of, 26
    conversion of, 31
    production of, 25, 29
estriol, chemical formula of, 26
estrogen
    function of, 77
    role in menstrual cycle, 77–80
estrone, chemical formula of, 26

follow-up studies on pill-users, 66–7,
    71–4, 89–90, 91–3

galactorrhea, pill-related, 139–41
gossypol, 118
Greenblatt, Robert, 33, 69, 70

health education, 45–6
hormones, action of during menstrual
 cycle, 76–80
 see also steroids *and individual steroids*
hormone withdrawal bleeds, 83

infertility, 52
inhibition of ovulation rates, 134–6

life expectation, effect of pill on, 93–5
lipid levels, changes in, 66, 72, 141–3
low-dosage pills, 130–40, 143, 144–5

males, means of fertility control for,
 17–20, 117–18
Marker, Russell E., 11–12, 29–30
mass media, 56–7, 63
menstrual cycle, 77–80
mestranol, 35, 36
metabolic changes due to the pill, 66
'morning after' pills, 120–1
mortality in pill-users, 90, 99–100,
 106–8, 129, 130, 144
myocardial infarction, 71, 90, 93, 94,
 126, 128–30, 142–3

nitrofurans, 117
norethisterone
 clinical trials on, 33–6
 synthesis of, 31

'once a month' pills, 118–20, 121
oral contraceptive pill
 attitude of medical profession
  towards, 41, 63
 attitude of R. C. Church towards,
  35, 110–13
 availability of, 90, 94, 98, 104–5, 110
 biphasic, 131, 133, 145
 clinical history of, 69–74
 contra-indications for, 54–5, 98
 cost of, 116, 124
 dosage of, 36, 41, 69–74, 130–40, 144
 effectiveness of, 83–4
 formulation of, 36, 45, 53, 69–74, 87,
  125–6

long-term benefits of, 57, 90–108
long-term risks of, 12, 52–3, 56–7,
 90–108, 125–30, 144
low-dosage, 130–40, 143, 144–5
mechanism of action of, 63–6, 80–4
opinion surveys on, 47–54
origins of, 11–12, 29–37, 87
perceived advantages of, 53–4
perceived disadvantages of, 50–3
progestin-only, 125–6
public attitude towards, 42–3, 57, 59,
 63, 67, 88, 97–8, 109–10
safety of, 49–50, 63, 67–8, 70–4,
 89–108, 126–30, 142–3, 144–5
sequential, 70, 134–5
side-effects of, 37, 42, 54, 70–3, 125,
 131, 136
 irreversible, 52–3
 reversible, 50–1
sources of information on, 54–9
triphasic, 74, 133–4, 135–7, 140–1,
 143, 145

package inserts, 57–8, 90
'paper' pills, 123
physiological changes due to the pill,
 63–6
'pill scares', 56, 63, 72, 73–4
Pincus, Gregory, 33–4
prescribing doctor, role of, 43, 55–6,
 104–6
production costs, 124
product liability, 58, 86, 116, 123, 124
progesterone
 chemical formula of, 26
 function of, 24, 79
 role of in menstrual cycle, 79–80
 synthesis of, 11–12, 25, 27–8, 31
progestin potency, 137, 139
prostaglandins, 119–20
Puerto Rico trials, 34, 36, 69, 89

quinestrol, 121

Rock, John, 33–35, 110–11
RU 486, 119

Searle, 33–6
sequential pills, 70, 134–5
sexual behaviour, changes in due to the
    pill, 42–3, 45
side-effects of the pill, 50–3
smoking, 53, 56, 71, 93–4, 97, 98, 100,
    107, 108, 128–9, 142, 144
steroids
    chemical formulae of, 26
    contraceptive, pharmacokinetics of,
        64–5, 72
    conversion of, 31
    function of, 23–4, 65
synthesis of, 25–8, 29–31, 33
stroke, 90, 93, 94, 142–3, 144
subdermal implants, 122–3
Syntex, 28, 30, 33, 35–6

testosterone
    chemical formula of, 26
    conversion of, 29, 31
    function of, 24
    synthesis of, 25, 30
    used as sperm suppressor, 117–18
thrombo-embolism, 53, 55, 71, 90,
    126–8, 130, 142, 144
thrombosis, 71–2, 89–90, 126–8
triphasic pills, 133–4, 135–7, 140–1,
    143, 145
Tyler, Edward, 33

vaginal rings, 123
venereal diseases, 109–10

yam, Mexican, 11, 26, 28, 29, 30